BIOLOGY OF THE
BRAIN

HOW YOUR GUT MICROBIOME
AFFECTS YOUR BRAIN

KENT MACLEOD R.Ph. B.Sc. Phm.

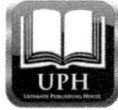

THE ULTIMATE PUBLISHING HOUSE (UPH) US HEADQUARTERS
P.O. Box 1204, Cypress, Texas, U.S.A. 77410

Canadian Office: 205 Glen Shields Avenue, Toronto, Ontario, Canada
L4K 2B0 Telephone: 647-883-1758

www.ultimatepublishinghouse.com
E-mail: info@ultimatepublishinghouse.com
www.BiologyoftheBrain.com

www.ultimatepublishinghouse.com
E-mail: info@ultimatepublishinghouse.com

US OFFICE: Ordering Information

Quantity Sales: COMPANIES, ORGANIZATIONS, INSTITUTIONS, AND INDUSTRY PUBLICATIONS.

Quantity discounts are available on bulk purchases of this book for reselling, educational purposes, subscription incentives, gifts, sponsorship, or fundraising. Unique books or book excerpts can also be fashioned to suit special needs such as private labeling with your logo on the cover and a message from or a message printed on the second page of the book. For more information, please contact our Special Sales Department at Ultimate Publishing House. Orders for college textbook or course adoption use.
Please contact Ultimate Publishing House Tel: 647-883-1758

ISBN: 978-1-7325389-3-1

BIOLOGY OF THE
BRAIN

HOW YOUR GUT MICROBIOME
AFFECTS YOUR BRAIN

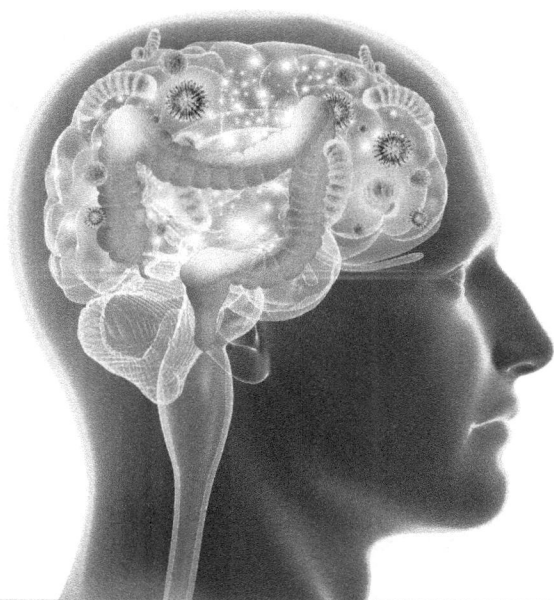

KENT MACLEOD R.Ph. B.Sc. Phm.
Foreword by Suzanne Somers

DEDICATION

I want to dedicate this book to Linda Pollon, my wife and life partner. She has always shone the light on my darkest corners. Without her light I would never have found a way forward.

ACKNOWLEDGEMENTS

My thought processes have always been in terms of molecules and chemistry. For this reason I have made it my practice to simply just tell people what they need to do, what they need to take, always using the best science. That entailed blurring the lines between natural and non-natural approaches trying to get to the root causes of disease.

While this sounds simple, it is anything but. I have needed a virtual army to support the scientific, psychological, existential, and business challenges on this journey. This Acknowledgement is but a token of gratitude for all those that have believed in me.

First of all, to my wife, Linda Pollon. For her to do the right thing is as normal as breathing. She would expect no less from me. She sets the bar for a high standard that I hope I can always achieve. She quiets my fears and embraces my hopes.

To Adam Livingston, who is tomorrow's visionary pharmacist here today. Without his endless hard work and dedication this book would never have been possible.

To my Italian mother-in-law, Yvette, who provided crucial no nonsense advice always cutting to the root of the matter.

To my children Kate, Emma, Andrew and Sophie. It scares me to think that I have inspired them to choose a similar path. On the other hand, it gives me such hope and inspiration that ultimately we are working for a better future.

To my parents John and Shirley for always being there for me and my family and supporting my work in any way they could.

To Dr. Abe Hoffer, Stephen Carter, Jonathan Prousky, Ron Hunnyhake, Rosalie Moscoe and all involved with the Orthomolecular Medicine Society and Canadian Schizophrenic Foundation.

For decades I have been part of this Society and observed relentless passion and dedication to finding "root" causes of mental health in spite of continuous criticism. The fact that their approaches were safe and effective and yet fell on deaf ears should inspire those in health care to improve and make a substantial impact on our health care system. This group gave me professional courage and perspective that sustained me for years.

So many doctors and health professionals have chosen this path less taken. They have gone against the grain and refused to prescribe unproven and risky medications.

Libuse Gilka, Bryn Waern, Joyce Buckley come to mind.

So many researchers continue to toil in obscurity knowing that finding root causes of disease will never have the same impact as finding the next new drug. We all rest on their shoulders.

To my tennis coaches and friends, Dale Power and Zhenya Kondratovski.

We always have agreed that anything you need in life could be learned on a tennis court.

Just keep the ball "over the net and between the lines".

I have also been fortunate to have met and been inspired by remarkable business people:

To Glen Luckman and Brent Wilson, the creators of Dymon Storage, my business partners for almost 25 years. They have shown me that honesty, integrity, focus, working hard, and doing what you believe in will always lead to success in business.

To a new wave of Nutritionists, Pharmacists, Naturopathic doctors and professionals that are also leading-"pushing" me to new exciting visions of the future:

Tanya Manikkam, Emma Pollon-MacLeod, Adam Livingston, Grace Meehan, Julia Davies, Kate Orlando, Laura Mierzwa, Kate Pollon-MacLeod.

Employees

I have two amazing people who have worked with me for over 35 years:

Lois Carroll, colleague, chemist, managing director of our compounding facility and dispensary. We have walked on many untraveled paths together, oftentimes with humour. She shared my passion and drive using science and chemistry to design natural products to improve people's lives.

Joyce Beveridge, my first employee. She worked with me since I was 24 years old. She taught me that integrity, humour and doing the right thing is what really matters in the end.

Suzanne Somers.

So many of my clients would come to see me clutching your books. You inspired them to seek me out, find a better way and not accept the status quo. This talent and dedication combined with your passion and caring allows people like me to be heard—thank you.

To my publisher, Felicia Pizzonia, who's enthusiasm and insistence that this could be done, inspired me to start and complete this project.

And finally, to my 40 years of wonderful, loyal clients who have trusted NutriChem implicitly with their health. Your unwavering support has inspired me to write this book. I thank you.

TABLE OF CONTENTS

FOREWORD
BY SUZANNE SOMERS

"The Biology of the Brain" How Your Gut Microbiome Affects Your Brain by Kent MacLeod, R.Ph. B.Sc. Phm. Is a Must Read!

Everyone has stomach issues. All I hear from my readers is "I'm bloated, I have stomach cramping, I'm constipated, I have terrible gas, I have unexplained weight gain". It goes on and on.

As we age, we encounter so many health problems, from bacterial overgrowth to inflammation, SIBO, (small intestinal bacterial overgrowth), that's your bloated intestines, to acid reflux with more and more people reporting esophageal cancer probably as a result of acid reflux. Acid reflux, otherwise known as GERD, (gastroesophageal reflux disease) is rampant. You see it in the swollen and irritated bellies of so many people causing terrible discomfort.

Personally, I too have been plagued by GI issues for the past several years. For me, It all started with a misdiagnosis, a nightmare so terrifying I have written about in two of my books. I was given 24-hour IV antibiotics for six days straight, night and day, medicine pouring into my veins for an infection I didn't have.

Little did I know this antibiotic invasion of my body would upset the microbiome in my GI tract for years to come and it's never been right since. In fact, at that time, I didn't even know what a microbiome was let alone try to fix it. I had no idea of gut balance and that gut balance was the right ratio of good bacteria to bad bacteria, yet here I was taking IV antibiotics that were taking away all balance. How was that going to make me healthy? I had no idea that the gut and the brain were so intertwined, so interconnected.

Neither did any of my doctors. No one told me that antibiotics "take away' (anti) and probiotics (pro) put back. Just that knowledge could have helped me avoid years of discomfort and unexplained weight gain. Simple probiotic replacement would have helped me rebalance.

There wasn't a definitive instructive book. Until this one.

I met Kent MacLeod several years ago when I was invited to Canada to lecture on behalf of his company NutriChem Pharmacy & Biomedical Clinic on bioidentical hormone replacement. I eagerly accepted, excited to introduce women and men in Canada to the joys of bioidentical hormone balance, a non-drug individualized natural hormone replacement protocol that puts back what you've lost in the aging process.

I was impressed that Kent MacLeod was so versed and knowledgeable about bioidenticals but also his vast knowledge of the body 'system' and that there is a language, a communications system so sophisticated that it puts any computer or technology to shame. When all is well, the system is called healthy and balanced, but how many people in today's world can call themselves truly healthy? If your gut is imbalanced you are not healthy, if that is so then you can bet that your brain is taking a hit also.

The gut and the brain are connected by a highway of sorts that I call the Vagus highway, (after the all-important Vagus nerve). Kent MacLeod will get more technical but I believe in visuals. This 'highway' goes from the gut to the brain and back at all times. Any interruption of the flow between these two important highways and you've got trouble. These two systems interact and communicate with one another constantly and that's why in the biggest picture, the interaction between the' gut and the brain' run the show.

This book by Kent Macleod explains this interaction in a way that is utterly understandable and gives the readers page after page of 'aha' moments.

We all want to know what's wrong and how to fix it. It's here in this book. You'll find In chapter after chapter that another 'light bulb' goes off and your understanding becomes deeper.

You will see yourself in this book. It will be the first time for many of you that it all starts to make sense.

Imagine a life with no bloating, no discomfort, fitting into your clothes, and on the other side, imagine a life with no more senior moments, forgetfulness, no autoimmune (yes autoimmune starts in the gut and then affects your brain); think fibromyalgia, Lupus, MS (multiple sclerosis), ADD (attention deficit), ADHD, OCD (obsessive compulsive disorder), depression, dyslexia, dyspraxia, autism, dementia, Alzheimer's and more. Imagine you could be well again and not reliant on a tackle box of drugs all causing side effects creating a need for more drugs. Its the merry-go-round of today.

Get off the carousel. You can fix yourself by reading this book.

Kent MacLeod tells you what is wrong, what you need, where to get it, how to do it and how to fix it.

Diet is crucial. Crucial. Imagine your body is a Maserati, the finest car in the world. You'd never put inferior fuel into a Maserati. Yet, look at how we all have been guilty of abusing our bodies by feeding ourselves inferior fuel. Our body is the greatest creation (machine) of all time.

We are lucky to now have access to the knowledge of healing and wellness.

This book will change your life.

"I believe that Nature is very intelligent.

The relationship between naturopathic medicine, clinical chemistry and pharmacy is divine when respecting nature.

Only when you respect Nature can you begin to understand it and unlock its healing power..."

— **Kent Macleod**

INTRODUCTION

"Every person takes the limits
of their own field of vision
for the limits of the world."

— Arthur Schopenhauer

What if I told you that there is a newly discovered organ?

What if I told you that it is comparable in size to your brain– roughly 2-3 lbs.?

This organ has the capability to communicate directly with your central nervous system, digestive tract, and it can stimulate the release of neurotransmitters, inflammatory markers, influence digestion and hormone levels – much like other organs in your body.

This organ is known as the microbiome. Think of it more as a virtual organ, rather than the classic image of a solid organ such as our liver or kidneys.

This is more of a futuristic organ, and it operates covertly – much like cloud-based storage. It is interconnected with everything. We know this organ is there, yet we cannot see it.

Sorry to be the one to tell you, but you do have this organ.
WE ALL DO.

This microscopic world within our bodies holds the potential to redefine how we understand disease, brain health, and ourselves.

Just as over time we have come to realize that the earth is not the center of our universe, and that we are orbiting just one of trillions of other stars, we are now coming to realize that humans are not the central inhabitants of our own bodies. Now is the time of the microbiome- even within ourselves, we are not the masters of our domain. We are made up of trillions of other living organisms that make us who we are.

In fact, if you look at it purely from a genetic standpoint – we have over 100 times more genetic material in our body from microbes than we do from human cells. We are outnumbered by our own microbes within us!

Would you think it's insane if I told you that we completely ignored this organ? …That we do not factor this organ into our healthcare?

The problem, as I see it, is not ignorance. We now know that the gut microbiome plays a vital role in our health. It's not the lack of knowledge, but the inability and unwillingness to change our views. We're animals of habit, and due to fear or comfort, we blind ourselves to necessary change and satisfy ourselves with the status quo. But what if that status quo is killing you?

I speak of limited beliefs, but this issue runs deeper than just limiting beliefs. It is a biochemistry problem. Processed foods full of sugar, preservatives, chemicals, as well as drugs, actually manipulate your gut bacteria and hijack your brain's pleasure centers to addict your brain to these substances.

People are not aware of how their microbiome and brain chemistry are being manipulated by processed foods and drugs. Even if I explain to a patient that these chemicals are very harmful for their microbiome and their health, and they believe it, this is not enough to help them necessarily. We must re-establish their microbiome.

We know that the gut microbiome affects the brain's development significantly. If this is an agreed upon notion, then why aren't we taking further action to introduce an infrastructure around *good* food and vitamins? The microbiome is still not respected as a significant contributor to brain development and mental health.

You can probably tell that I'm a little obsessed with this subject. This infatuation began many years ago, but my real "ah-ha" moment, which prompted the writing of this book, took place when I attended an addiction conference in Calgary, Alberta, Canada.

The keynote speaker was explaining how a 100 million-dollar program could convince professionals to grasp the concept that early childhood experiences affect the biological structure of the brain. The more adverse experiences you have early in life, the greater the risk of physical and mental health issues later in life.

The doctors here were stuck in the old way of thinking. They discussed how early-life neglect negatively impacted the brain, but there was no mention of the gut microbiome and its vital importance to the body's overall health. I was the only one talking about it. Within the category of neglect, we can find nutritional neglect, but this was only being mentioned as a footnote, while it should have been at the forefront of every discussion.

I found myself thinking, "What if we introduced the principle of the importance of nutrition and the microbiome? How would that alter the course of their lives in a positive way?"

I actually began to laugh during the conference. Not the joy-filled laugh, but one of incredulous shock. Here we were about to spend millions training and educating people about the structure of the brain and what affects it, without any mention of nutrition and the microbiome?!

I had always tried to be a part of the conversation and share what I had learned over the last thirty-five years about the interconnection between the brain and the gut, but this conference showed me I had not gotten as far as I had hoped.

If there was one thing this conference revealed to me, it was that we still had a long way to go.

Regularly, I see patients who will not change their diet even though they know it would be good for them, because they are addicted. This is the purpose of these industries. It is a perfect symbiosis between big food and big pharma. It is a multibillion dollar industry. People are diseased because of junk food, and then they require drugs to treat the diseases from eating junk food.

"Brain health is microbiome health."

— Kent MacLeod

If we look throughout the history and development of medicine, we'll see the same thing. Since my graduation from pharmacy school thirty-five years ago, we're still doing and saying the same things we were decades ago. We use basically the same drugs but expect different results.

We've pumped tens of millions of dollars into the mental health epidemic but have failed to address root causes. Very often, people don't just have mental health conditions, they also have a *malnourished microbiome, crying out for help.*

If I had unlimited time, I'd teach this throughout the world until everyone understood the importance of their guts. The facts, the evidence, and the research is all there and self-evident. My goal is not to eliminate modern medicine, but to use it for what it does best: acute care.

It's a slow process, but I firmly believe most doctors and medical professionals mean well. They have good intentions, but intentions are useless if you don't take action. To go one step further, ineffective action is worse than good intentions. These professionals are discouraged from exploring alternative medicinal sources and strategies because it doesn't fall within the scope of the current medical guidelines.

From the moment we opened our doors at NutriChem, we've never wavered in our belief that continued growth, development, and learning is key to medical progress. We've held numerous seminars and webinars that medical professionals have attended and engaged in the debate on gut health.

I'm encouraged to see more and more professionals taking an interest in and implementing these new truths about the gut microbiome and its effect on our health.

The biology of the brain begins in the gut.

And so, begins our journey…

CHAPTER 1

THE MICROBIOME AND WHAT IT MEANS FOR YOU

"All disease starts in the gut."

— Hippocrates, The Father of Medicine

You rush to the bathroom for the tenth time in as many minutes. You can't seem to shake the diarrhea or the throbbing pain in your stomach. You think back to your last meal and shake your head. Maybe you shouldn't have eaten that cheeseburger. The meat must have been bad, or the cheese, or the lettuce. Maybe the cook didn't wash his hands.

Your stomach buckles and you forget about the numerous possibilities that might have caused your current predicament. Your throat contracts suddenly. You barely make it to your knees before the flash flood of bile, food, and water heave up your esophagus and pour into the toilet. Why are you so sick?

Do you have the flu or just the twenty-four-hour bug?

God, you hope so! You can't take another day of this and you're only in the first hour.

You cling to the toilet with both hands until the sixth upheaval that feels like a small rodent is burrowing its way out of your chest stops. Your head flops forward in surrender. Your chest rises and falls in quick succession as you take in gulps of air to avert the nausea already swelling in your tummy.

Your body is shaking, you're sweating, and you feel weak. You flush then rinse out your mouth in the sink and go back to bed. You don't make it ten feet before you rush back to the toilet.

Does this story sound familiar?

Perhaps you struggle with chronic diarrhea, vomiting, cramping, pain, hot and cold flashes, migraines, fatigue, trouble sleeping or concentrating, inability to complete tasks, or fear of leaving your home without a toilet nearby, and any number of *normal* ailments that affect people every day.

Doctors might diagnose you with an anxiety disorder, an allergy, or irritable bowel syndrome (IBS), and then prescribe you medications to *fix* your disorder. But your health problems are only getting worse, and recently, more irregularities are showing up. You've been subjected to what seems like hundreds of tests, blood work, scans of your body and brain, and even seen multiple psychiatrists or specialists. Nothing seems to work.

The doctors ensure you that you're on the right track to recovering and to *stick to the process*. But your gut tells you that something else is wrong. Your gut tells you that they haven't gotten to the bottom of the problem.

"Never apologize for trusting your intuition—your brain can play tricks, your heart can be blind, but your gut is always right."

— Rachel Wolchin

If the doctors and the supposed specialists can't figure out what's wrong with you and only seem to make matters worse, is there any hope for you ever recovering and getting your life back?

Yes, but it begins by understanding the root cause of your distress: the gut.

Oh, and by the way, when I refer to "the gut," I am referring to the entire digestive system.

THE MICROBIOME

Some of you might be thinking, "What the heck is a microbiome? Is that like one of those shelters on Mars, used to terraform the red planet?" While I enjoy the idea of man making Mars suitable for survival, it's not my specialty.

I deal primarily with facts and proven science.

In my thirty-five plus years in the pharmaceutical industry, I've learned two things. One, science is ever-changing. And two, sometimes we're wrong.

Both are true in the case of the microbiome.

Modern medicine still claims to be the answer to all of your health problems: mental, physical, and emotional.

Just take this pill and you'll feel better. And for a time, this proves true. But then the real monster rears its head. You're sicker than you've ever been before, and those same doctors, operating in a fog have the same solution: more pills.

As you go around and round in this never-ending cycle of medication, with no healing in sight, you're trapped in a realm of desperation and helplessness. But you don't need to be and you shouldn't have to settle for mediocre science and traditional ways of thinking about health.

At NutriChem, we specialize in honing in on the root problem for any and all of your health issues. And time and time again, we find that there's a direct correlation between your symptoms and an unstable, compromised, or damaged gut microbiome.

WHAT IS YOUR GUT MICROBIOME?

The gut microbiome is a two-to-five-pound biomass comprised of bacteria, fungi, and other microorganisms that primarily reside in the large intestine. It is the collection of microorganisms throughout your entire gastrointestinal tract. The stomach has distinct bacteria that tend to occupy it, the small intestine has distinct bacteria that tend to occupy it, and the large intestine has the highest concentration of bacteria that occupy it. When we refer generally to "the microbiome", we are typically referring to the large intestinal microbiome because it is the "headquarters" microbiome with the most bacteria of any organ in the body; however, there are many microbiomes (e.g. the skin, the gut, the vagina, etc.).

There are thousands of different species of bacteria that live in your gut. These are what are known as both good and bad bacteria. Naturally, you want to increase the number of good bacteria in your gut, as this stimulates a healthy and balanced gastrointestinal system. Adversely, if the number of bad bacteria increase, this is where the problems come in.

The microbiome is a complex ecosystem like a forest.

Picture a tropical rainforest.

Just think of a rainforest with four main plant structures e.g. trees, shrubs, grasses, and vines, for example- they all rely on each other for optimal survival. A healthy forest needs all four groups of plants to thrive. If one is missing, the structure of the whole forest is compromised.

There are general structures (e.g. trees or shrubs)- these are called phylum. Within these major groups or phyla, there are specific species. Some people with major health issues are lacking entire phyla of bacteria, whereas other people are only missing a few species within these phyla.

The trees or shrubs are not standalone entities. They branch out and connect with other trees and plants in the ecosystem around it. Just as its roots interconnect through the soil beneath it, so too does your microbiome connect with your environment.

When it comes to the microbiome, you can't miss the forest for the trees!

We often take a reductionist approach and aim to look at one species of bacteria, but it is the entire larger ecosystem that is important! See the bigger picture.

No one species is self-independent. We are all interdependent on the other. Cause an imbalance in one, and another will become compromised. If you remove a group or species, the ecosystem is imbalanced and disturbed. Take away the rain and other biomass in the forest that provides food for the soil, and the soil loses its potency for the plants that grow in it.

Think of your microbiome as a rainforest- its plants, animals, soil, and canopy- the entire ecosystem. Just as its roots spread out into the soil and its branches stretch toward the sun, your microbiome connects to different parts of your body on a molecular level.

THE MAKEUP OF THE MICROBIOME

"There are few things in life that are as fascinating and challenging as understanding the inextricable connection between our microbiome and our brain."

— Kent MacLeod, founder of NutriChem

The gut is its own ecosystem, much like any other ecosystem in the world. Within each system lies an array of moving parts that each have a unique role to play. Your human body can survive without an arm or a leg, but you become less effective as a whole. The same goes for any ecosystem; it may still appear to function, but it is compensating for and suffering as a result of the missing or damaged parts.

The problem comes when you either take away or damage some moving parts or hinder one that controls the rest. Think of it as the heart or brain of the system. Without it, nothing else functions.

The gut microbiome consists of four primary groups of bacteria.

- Firmicutes
- Bacteroidetes
- Actinobacteria
- Proteobacteria

NUTRICHEM'S *MICROBIOME MAP*

"Keystone" Bacterial Group	Preferred Fiber/Prebiotic "Fuel Source"

1. Actinobacteria
 	
Species:
• *Bifidobacterium Longum*
• *Bifidobacterium Lactis*
• *Bifidobacterium Infantis*
• *Bifidobacterium Bifidum*
	Fructans (oligosaccharides and polysaccharides)
	
	Food Sources:
	Onions, leeks, garlic, artichokes, chicory, asparagus, fruits (pomegranates, agave, bananas), cereals, grains (wheat, barley, spelt)
	
	Supplement Sources:
	    • FOS
	    • GOS
	    • XOS
	    • IMO
	    • Inulin

2. Firmicutes
 	
a. Clostridia Cluster IV
 	
Species:
• *Faecalibacterium prausnitzii*
	Pectins
	
	Food Sources:
	*Citrus fruits (oranges, limes, lemons), pears, apples, plums, carrots
	
	Supplement Sources:
	    • Modified Citrus Pectin
	    • Fractionated Pectin Powders
	    • Apple Pectins
	    • Bioflavonoids from citrus peels

THE BIOLOGY OF THE BRAIN

• *Ruminococcus bromii*	**Resistant Starch** Food Sources: Oats, rices, legumes, cashews, wheat bran/bran cereals, cooled potato starch Supplement Sources: Raw, unmodified potato starch
b. Clostridia Cluster XIVa **Species:** • *Roseburia intestinalis*	**Fructans** (oligosaccharides and polysaccharides) Food Sources: Onions, leeks, garlic, artichokes, chicory, asparagus, fruits (pomegranates, agave, bananas, etc.), cereals, grains (wheat, barley, spelt) Supplement Sources: • FOS • GOS • XOS • IMO • Inulin
• *Eubacteria rectate*	**Inulin** Food Sources: Chicory root, dandelion, asparagus, garlic, leeks, onions, bananas, plantains, Ezekiel bread (sprouted wheat) Supplement Sources: Inulin Fiber (most often from chicory root)

3. Bacteroidetes	
• *Bacteroides vulgatus*	**Inulin, fat** Inulin Food Sources: Chicory root, dandelion, asparagus, garlic, leeks, onions, bananas, plantains, Ezekiel bread (sprouted wheat) Inulin Supplement Sources: - Inulin Fiber (most often from chicory root)
• *Alistipes putredinis*	**Lignins** Food Sources: Whole grains, wheat bran, corn bran, legumes, nuts, seeds, potato skins, lignans (polyphenols in many plants and foods), many vegetables, avocado, unripe bananas

NutriChem's Microbiome Map is a system we use at our integrative healthcare center to classify important "good" bacterial strains, or "keystone species", required for a healthy microbiome, as well as the types of fibers that must be ingested to increase levels of these good bacteria in the large intestine.

I know. I'm sure you use these terms on a daily basis with your friends and kids. While these may not be normal household names, the key takeaway is that most microbial bacteria belong to these four phyla.

Just so you know...

I'll be using terms throughout this book that you may have heard of, be familiar with, or may be hearing for the first time. I'll do my best to explain each one, where needed, but will focus on why they matter and what they mean for you.

Each one of these groups is crucial for an effective gut microbiome. And each one serves its own purpose. Much like each soldier within a combat unit specializes in their own task, each one works together for the same fight or battle.

There's a distinct correlation between an imbalance in any one of these bacteria groups to things like obesity, addiction, pain, depression, anxiety, various other mental health issues, and gastrointestinal problems. Imbalances in these bacterial groups can inflame your gut and brain.

Our goal is to determine what those imbalances are and how to correct them. However, this requires specialized testing that most medical professionals either are unwilling to perform or don't consider when diagnosing a patient.

Most professionals only examine the brain and not the gut. This should be the other way around.

In addition to the required testing to locate any imbalance, there are also practical ways to self-examine your body to determine if there's a potential microbiome imbalance. The purpose of this book is to give you the tools to understand your body and take the necessary steps to function at your optimal level.

I am aware that what I'll teach you is not a mainstream practice or theory. The G.U.T. Theory is the premise that all of this is based on and this theory flips all medical theories on their heads and completely transforms how we look at medicine, the body, the mind, and the gut.

G.U.T. Theory

The Grand Unified Theory (or G.U.T Theory) of health is the concept that the human body can be viewed as one vessel with multiple systems that are all influenced by a single, underlying central router: the microbiome.

Cutting-edge research has shown that many mental health patients are missing one or more of the four primary bacterial groups. This is no coincidence. The gut can be a fundamental source of health or sickness.

While many practitioners may be resistant to change, they cannot refute the results of addressing the process that leads to a healthier microbiome. I believe in following the facts and evidence. Throughout this book, I will share case studies of patients whom I've helped to overcome, reduce, or completely eradicate addictions, hypertension, anxiety, depression, obesity, low energy levels, insomnia, memory loss, lack of focus and concentration, IBS, migraines, chronic pain, and many such symptoms or ailments that affect most people around the globe on a daily basis.

If you're someone who suffers from one of the health problems listed or something similar, there's a very good chance that the cause is a damaged or imbalanced microbiome. I'm committed to helping you find the root cause of your discomfort and remove it so that you can begin living the life that you were meant to live.

Myself and my team at NutriChem have helped thousands of patients restore their health through their microbiomes. These mothers, fathers, sons, daughters, business men and women, friends, coworkers, and strangers on the street are people just like you and me who finally found the truth and took action.

They now live life to the fullest. Once their microbiomes were restored, they found that it takes little effort to maintain that newfound balance. If you're ready to regain control of your life, start living the way you were meant to, and reduce, improve, or completely wipe out your health problems (without taking a bucket of pills and spending thousands on medical visits), then continue reading as we dive into the top eight connections between the gut and the brain.

MICROFLORA FACT:

You inherit your microbiome from your mother during the birth process. The mother-to-child transference of microflora depends on the type of birth: vaginal versus C-section. This can create differences in the child's microbiome that are associated with long-term autoimmunity, asthma, eczema, and obesity.

THE GUT-BRAIN AXIS: THE TOP EIGHT WAYS YOUR GUT AND YOUR BRAIN COMMUNICATE

Now that we understand what the microbiome is, let's delve into how our environment, and what we eat or do affect either the disruption or sustainability of our microbiomes.

Just as higher levels of *firmicutes* with decreased levels of *bacteroidetes* are linked to obesity and inflammation, there are direct correlations in the changes or fluctuations of the microbiome in other physical, emotional, and psychological disorders.

While diet plays a more important role in microbiome health than you may even know, we'll discuss diet and its effect on the microbiome more in Chapter 7.

For the purposes of this section, we'll focus our attention on the top eight connections that take place between the gut and brain.

Picture these as the top eight ways that your microbiome can influence your brain.

Throughout this book, you'll hear more about each of these connections in greater depth as they pertain to specific health problems.

THE TOP EIGHT WAYS YOUR GUT AND YOUR BRAIN COMMUNICATE:

- The Vagus Nerve
- Cortisol
- Neurotransmitters (e.g. serotonin)
- Neuropeptides (gut hormones)
- Absorption, metabolism, and activation of nutrients and minerals
- Sex hormone disruption
- Bacterial strains
- Drugs (over-the-counter, prescribed, or abused substances)

Let's break each one of these down in layman's terms, explore their roles in the body, and examine how they affect the microbiome.

The Vagus Nerve

This is your brain's physical connection to your gut.

The vagus nerve holds multiple responsibilities within the body. Think of it as a multi-level freeway that links the gut and the brain.

It handles sensory processes for the throat, heart, lungs, and abdomen (gut). It also provides sensations for taste due to its connection on the back of the tongue. In addition, its motor functions help you to swallow or speak.

For the purpose of this book, we will focus on its primary feature, which is sending information between the brain and the gut. The gut is directly linked to the handling of stress, anxiety, and fear.

Ever wonder why some people get nervous diarrhea before a presentation? Or butterflies in the stomach? It's the vagus nerve. When your body senses fear or stress, it activates the vagus nerve, which has an impact on the gut.

The vagus nerve is like a switch between your body's sympathetic (fight or flight) and parasympathetic (rest and digest) systems. When stressed, adrenaline activates the vagus nerve and causes release of cortisol in the gut. Too much cortisol in the gut, over time, such as with chronic stress, damages it. And a damaged gut, in turn, can cause stress and anxiety via the vagus nerve. It is a two-way street.

When left untreated, it'll cause inflammation and damage the gut's microbiome.

Cortisol

Commonly referred to as the "stress hormone", cortisol is a steroid hormone produced by the adrenal cortex and plays a role in metabolizing carbohydrates and proteins.

Cortisol is the main hormone involved in the HPA axis. It's known for handling the body's stress response, but holds other important roles as well.

It is also highly involved in regulating blood sugar levels, metabolism, inflammation, memory formation, salt and water equilibrium, as well as blood pressure.

While cortisol is seen as a hindrance to the body, it actually is a key ingredient to the body's well-being. The only problem is when there are chronic high levels of this hormone in the body. This in turn disrupts the gut microbiome and can be responsible for weight gain, anxiety, and depression.Chronic stress leads to chronic cortisol release in the gut, which causes damage to the gastrointestinal tract and microbiome. Long-term stress and resulting high cortisol damages the microbiome. This damage to the microbiome can contribute to mental illness.

Anyone with a gut condition such as inflammatory bowel disease or irritable bowel syndrome knows that when they go through a stressful time in their lives, their condition worsens or "flairs" for a short period of time. This is due to increased cortisol during stressful periods, which harms the microbiome and worsens gastrointestinal diseases, as well as mental health conditions.

But remember, the communication is bi-directional, so having certain strains of bacteria in the gut can make people more or less sensitive to stress. So, if you have a lot of unhealthy bacteria in your gut, a minor stress will result in a major cortisol release, compared to a gut with healthy bacteria that is more resilient and less reactive to stressors. This has been shown in mice studies, where they stress mice out with healthy guts versus unhealthy guts and also in studies where they can transplant the gut bacteria of anxious versus relaxed mice into each other and watch their behavior switch. Mice with bad gut bacteria showed much more anxious behaviors than mice with healthy guts in many studies.

With the modern day doctor pouring medication over the problem, you can see how the root cause is easily overlooked and more problems are caused by mistreating the illness. The answer is not always medication. It's microbiome restoration.

Neurotransmitters (serotonin, dopamine, norepinephrine, etc.)

Serotonin is the main focus here. It is commonly referred to as the "happy" or "feel good" neurotransmitter.

When we think of serotonin, we often think about the brain, but did you know that…

Nearly 90% of serotonin is produced in the gut. Antidepressants are a multi-billion-dollar industry, which manipulate serotonin levels in the brain. The problem is that it seldom offers lasting results without increasing the dosage of the drug continuously.

The body uses serotonin as a messenger (neurotransmitter) between nerve cells. It regulates functions such as mood, behavior, appetite, digestion, sleep, memory, and sex. Altering serotonin levels has been used to treat people with depression and anxiety, or those who suffer from chronic migraines, nausea, and even combat obesity.

Most antidepressant drugs, known as selective serotonin reuptake inhibitors (SSRIs), work by increasing levels of serotonin between brain cells. SSRI drugs aim to redistribute serotonin, not synthesize or replenish it, and they are poorly effective with many side effects. They only redistribute serotonin instead of producing it, and therefore, often stop working over time and require higher doses.

The manufacture and distribution of serotonin to the brain is proven to be regulated by the gut.

If you believe in SSRI drugs for depression because you believe in the serotonin hypothesis of depression, then you should know about the science of serotonin and its essential connection to the gut! Availability of serotonin to the brain is even regulated by the gut too! It is bizarre that we use drugs to boost serotonin, but we don't look at the biggest producer of serotonin in the body- the gut!

Drugs damage the gut, which in turn impairs the body's natural production of this neurotransmitter.

In mice studies, those with disrupted microbiomes produced significantly less serotonin than those with healthy microbiomes.

Furthermore, certain antibiotics that affect gut bacteria are currently being explored and used for treatment of resistant depression (depression that does not respond to antidepressants).

A good way to think about the gut is like a well in the middle of a hot desert. The well has water at the base, but you have to use a pulley and bucket to retrieve it. The sun is beating down on you, you're sweating, and it's so hot that you could pass out.

Your body is quickly dehydrating. Your life depends on this water buried beneath the sand. But as you come up to the well, you notice that the bucket is gone and the pulley system is broken. There's no way to get to the water. You have one of three choices: find another way to get to the water, keep walking and hope you'll find another well, or do nothing.

All three are poor choices when the natural order of things was the pulley system with the bucket, but someone or something (environment) damaged them.

It is the same with the gut. It's the well of life for your body, but you can either poison the water or damage the systems (pulleys) that connect to it. This is what poor diet, prescribed medications, drugs, and the environment can do to your microbiome.

Neuropeptides

These are messenger molecules between the gut and brain. Neuropeptides communicate important messages such as hunger and satiety, and they are produced primarily in the gut.

These molecules influence how the brain communicates with the rest of the body, and if damaged, your brain will learn to respond in an unfavorable way.

Think of all of the areas that your brain is responsible for: food intake, metabolism, addictions (food & drug), reproduction, memory, learning, and social behavior.

The following are examples of neuropeptides that specifically involve or affect the gut:

- glucagon-like peptide-1 (GLP-1) — controls blood sugar levels and secreting insulin.
- cholecystokinin (CCK) — responsible for the digestion of fats and proteins.
- ghrelin — known as the "hunger hormone". It regulates the body's hunger response.
- leptin — known as the "anti-hunger hormone". It regulates energy by balancing hunger.

Let's look at obesity, for example. If you have malfunctioning hunger messages between your gut and brain, you will not feel the signal to stop eating. There is emerging evidence showing that an unhealthy microbiome is a risk factor for obesity, and it is believed to be via a neuropeptide signaling disruption. A disrupted microbiome leads to disrupted neuropeptide signaling, leading to disrupted hunger patterns and overeating.

Absorption, Metabolism, and Activation of Nutrients and Minerals

Optimal absorption of nutrients depends on a healthy microbiome. You could eat a healthy diet, but if your microbiome is disrupted, you will be unable to absorb the nutrients you consume. ALL ingested nutrients depend on the microbiome for proper metabolism and absorption.

Also, certain nutrients must be metabolized and activated in order to perform their biochemical functions. This too requires a healthy microbiome.

An important aspect of a healthy microbiome is sufficient and effective absorption, metabolizing of proteins and fats, and activation of nutrients and minerals.

Without these, your body will not perform at its prime capacity.

Some of the most important metabolites for gut health are known as short chain fatty acids, or *SCFAs*. SCFAs are produced primarily by gut bacteria digesting soluble fibers, or prebiotics, and they play key roles in protecting the gut lining, reducing gastrointestinal inflammation, and they also act as important signaling molecules on a variety of cells beyond the digestive system. A healthy gut, fed generous quantities of soluble prebiotic fibre, can produce large amounts of SCFAs like acetate, propionate, and butyrate. Generally, the more SCFAs your gut can produce, the healthier it will be.

The gut microbiome is also very important for prevention of nutrient deficiencies. Some of the most common nutrient deficiencies are iron, iodine, vitamin D, vitamin B12, vitamin B6, magnesium, and zinc. Only the gut can metabolize these, and only a healthy gut can activate them.

Vitamin B6 must be activated to its active form via a healthy microbiome. This fact, along with malnutrition, makes low vitamin B6 one of the most prevalent deficiencies in the world. The active form of Vitamin B6, known as P5P (pyridoxal-5-phosphate), is an effective treatment for several conditions such as nerve pain, neuropathy, PMS, water retention, depression, and seizures. A large portion of the world's population is deficient in Vitamin B6. Roughly 75% of young women (especially those on oral contraceptives), are deficient in B6. And B6 must be activated to P5P, so we must know about this activation and how vitamin B6 is activated!

Vitamin B6 is involved in over 140 biochemical reactions in the human body, including the synthesis of serotonin. If we go back to serotonin and its key benefits to the human body, B6 is also a key determinant in serotonin's production.

With much of the world deficient, there's a good chance that your microbiome is disrupted, even if you *feel* healthy. Oftentimes, a microbiome is damaged or compromised without the person knowing it. It's not until other ailments arise that you become aware of a microbiome disruption.

INTERESTING FACT:
Excessive alcohol consumption can lead to B-vitamin deficiencies. While doctors have noted that vitamin B6 is a key molecule for preventing alcoholic neuropathy and liver damage, no studies or research on addiction have done their due diligence to link these to a compromised gut microbiome.

In addition to B6, two other nutrients are vital for brain function, but are often absorbed or activated improperly. They are magnesium and iron.

Magnesium helps regulate hundreds of biochemical reactions in the body. Some of these include protein synthesis (creating something chemically), blood glucose control, blood pressure, and muscle & nerve function. Magnesium is one of THE most critical nutrients in the body. It also transports calcium and potassium ions through cell membranes, which is crucial for nerve impulse conduction, muscle contractions, and heart rhythms. It is involved in hundreds of processes and has more critical processes dependent upon it than any other essential nutrient!

Magnesium also plays a role in producing energy, as well as synthesizing DNA (the makeup of all cells in the body and responsible for life), RNA (DNA's messenger), and the structural development of bones.

Not all magnesium is created equal! Many magnesium salts, such as magnesium oxide and magnesium citrate, are poorly absorbed through the gut and have more of a laxative effect. Conversely, other magnesium salts, such as magnesium glycinate, bisglycinate, and threonate, absorb much more readily through the gastrointestinal tract and enter the bloodstream and cells much more easily. In patients with a compromised microbiome, highly absorbed magnesium salts are a better option. Unless you want a laxative effect, highly absorbable magnesium is a better choice for most patients.

Iron is a key component for the production of hemoglobin. Hemoglobin is the protein on red blood cells that is responsible for carrying oxygen from the lungs to the rest of the body.

Having the right amount of iron in your bloodstream is vital to your health. Have too little (anemia) and you might suffer from poor oxygen delivery to your tissues and low energy. This usually is found in patients with a diet low in iron or excessive bleeding during menstruation in women. Adversely, too much iron (hemochromatosis) is when your body stores too much iron. This can actually poison your body.

Many women know that absorbing adequate iron can be difficult. Many women suffer from low iron and anemia. Earlier in my career, I would try to give women higher doses of more potent iron with modest effects. However, when I started to correct the microbiome first, and then gave iron, their iron levels rose much more effectively, exhibiting the impact of the microbiome on iron absorption. This is important to note because there are studies showing that iron supplementation can actually disrupt the microbiome in some cases.

Sex Hormone Disruption

There is an established connection between sex hormones, the microbiome, and the brain.

You may not have realized, but your sex hormones play a more important role than just reproduction. Excessive cortisol in the bloodstream will impact your sex hormones, as well as your gut and overall health. Too much cortisol, without a balance, is associated with cancers, heart disease, mental health disorders, and many other medical conditions.

There is a cortisol connection to this and too much cortisol damages the microbiome.

In men, the stress hormone, cortisol, lowers testosterone.

In women, stress leads to production of cortisol from the hormone precursor DHEA, which is also required for production of progesterone. Therefore, increased cortisol leads to decreased progesterone, a female hormone required for proper sleep, relaxation, and fertility.

I'll touch more on hormones and their importance in Chapter 6 – Hormones.

Bacterial Strains

Bacteria is often seen as a bad thing. We're taught to wash our hands and not lick dirty objects because "there is bacteria on them." But this misconception is misleading.

Yes, there are bad bacteria and we want to minimize those in our intake, but there are also good bacteria that strengthen your immune system and other functions of your body.

When a microbiome is damaged, there's usually more bad bacteria than good. The good news is that this isn't permanent. You can restore a balanced microbiome with the right process. We'll talk more on this in the chapters dedicated to microbiome mapping (chapters 7-10).

So, what are considered healthy bacteria?

These are any bacteria that boost the body's immune system, improve digestion, and balance the microbiome, resulting in improvement of a number of chronic illnesses. They also combat bad bacteria that invade the gut.

For example, two good bacteria, bifidobacteria and lactobacteria strains, have been clinically proven to positively affect mood, anxiety, and stress. These also tie into cognitive and mental wellness. These strains are known as psychobiotics, primarily because they help with mood and behavior, even though we don't know yet why.

In addition, prebiotics, food for probiotics (think fiber), enhance the growth of good bacteria in the gut microbiome. These *feed* good bacteria. They're imperative for intestinal and brain health.

Approximately 80-90% of Canadians and Americans are fiber deficient. Fiber is crucial to anchor healthy probiotic bacteria in the gut. Other than fiber supplements, there are some foods you can eat to build a strong fiber intake.

Some include:

- chia seeds
- flaxseeds
- fruits (raspberries, blackberries, pears)
- vegetables (broccoli, peas, lima beans, lentils, split peas)
- sweet potatoes
- wheat germ
- black beans
- artichokes
- avocados
- bran flakes
- whole-wheat pasta
- oatmeal
- pearled barley
- raw chicory root
- raw Jerusalem artichoke
- raw garlic
- raw dandelion greens
- raw leeks
- raw onions

Here are fermented foods that are probiotic sources:

- apple cider vinegar
- fermented vegetables (kimchi, sauerkraut, natto)
- goat milk yogurt
- kefir

- coconut kefir
- kombucha
- kvass
- miso

Toxic Effects from Drugs

Many of the imbalances in the microbiome are a direct result of poor diet, medications, and toxic substances. These disrupt and destroy the microbiome, and create an environment for bad bacteria, diseases, and viruses to thrive.

This is by far the most damaging and dangerous of the influencers for the microbiome. Not only because of their affect on the body and its ecosystem, but because they are so easy to come by. It's almost like going to the store and buying candy.

Pharmacies and doctors hand out antibiotics, NSAIDS, and PPI drugs as though they are the most natural choice. Canada and America are amongst the most medicated nations in the world while also being the most obese and suffering from some of the highest rates of mental illnesses. We are also the #1 (US) and #3 (Canada) nations with the highest prescription drug spending per capita in the world.

We'll talk more on this in the next chapter, *Big Threats, Big Impact*.

Some of these eight influencers occur naturally in the body through your chemical or genetic makeup. However, many are a direct response to what you can control. And if you can control it, then you can tilt the scale in your favor and improve your health.

LET'S TALK "BLUE ZONES"

These are "longevity hotspots" around the world where people have the longest average lifespans and the highest rates of centenarian citizens (people who make it to age 100 or higher). But age is only one factor. They also maintain active cognitive and physical functions, and diseases like type 2 diabetes basically don't exist in these "blue zones." Not coincidentally, these "blue zone" inhabitants also have some of the healthiest lifestyles and healthiest microbiomes in the world.

As we know, diabetes correlates to a higher risk of cardiovascular disease, cancer, and basically every disease known to man. So, when diabetes is not present, it's only natural that other diseases would not exist either, which facilitates a higher functioning society. One of the biggest correlates of mental health disorder is diabetes. So naturally, the question is then asked, "Why doesn't diabetes exist in these populations?"

Whether it's North America, Europe, South America, or Asia where these blue zones exist, what is the "thing" that is unique about them? Some studies indicate that they all have and maintain healthier microbiomes, regardless of what they eat. But again, of course their diet is crucial to overall health and longevity and tends to coincide with more whole foods and less processed foods.

Someone else may argue that these blue zones exist due to their-lifestyles with more exercise, less stress, and social interactions. But all of those things have also been proven to help the microbiome.

The "Blue Zones" are:
1.   Loma Linda, California
2.   Nicoya, Costa Rica
3.   Sardinia, Italy
4.   Icaria, Greece
5.   Okinawa, Japan

Blue Zones/Longevity Hotspots

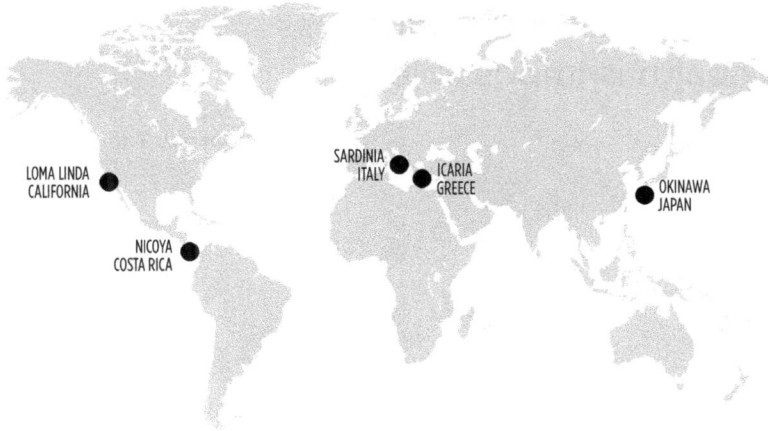

Blue Zone Life Lessons

- move naturally
- eat wisely
- right outlook
- right tribe

BRAIN POWER TIP

People are beginning to lean more toward holistic approaches to health and wellness. I believe this is the body's natural intuition bleeding through to awaken us to the real problems affecting our guts.

However, it's important to understand that medication, diet, or exercise is not enough. If your microbiome is disrupted, your brain cannot rewire itself. It would be like saying, "I'm going to be a better driver after I take this driving course" but your car has flat tires, no brakes, the battery's dead, and the windshield is cracked.

The underlying mechanism—your gut microbiome (or car in this example)—must be corrected FIRST to find true success and revive your health.

"In a disordered mind, as in a disordered body, soundness of health is impossible."

— Marcus Tullius Cicero

CHAPTER 2

THREATS TO YOUR MICROBIOME & HEALTHY LIVING

"We cannot assume whether any product is good or bad until we know what it does to the microbiome."

— Kent MacLeod

I'll never forget this 63-year-old woman who'd come into my clinic. We'll call her Susie. Susie had type two diabetes, suffered from obesity, and from severe high blood sugar. She tried diets and to exercise to lose the weight, but nothing worked.

She even resorted to medication to stimulate normal blood sugar levels and weight loss. This only made matters worse for her. By the time she came to me, she was desperate (it's unfortunate I was seen as the last resort, but I'm glad she came to me).

We evaluated her lifestyle, her food intake, her diet, her regimen, her medications. We went over her prior tests, then did our own full-body analysis to determine the culprit of her health issues and inability to lose weight.

Can you guess what it was?

You're right. Her gut microbiome was all out of whack and needed a drastic recovery if she had any hope of living an abundant life without worry, stress, and chronic health failure. After I went over the test results with her and explained her situation, she became noticeably distraught.

She had been struggling with her weight for years and she had made it her identity. She was never going to lose weight and would always have diabetes and health problems. There was no hope for her. As she wiped the tears from her eyes and lifted her head to me, I asked her one question, "Susie, do you want to get well?"

You might be thinking, "Jeez! Kent. Why don't you just slap the girl! Of course, she wants to get well!" Maybe you're right, but it's never quite so simple. You see, like Susie, many people around the world suffer from what I would call an "identity crisis". This is different than what you may have previously heard.

Instead, it runs deeper to the core of who we are as social beings. You see, Susie had become her health problems. She was no longer Susie, but her diabetes, her weight, her failures, her inability to sleep, her self-consciousness, her lack of engagement with the world, her low energy, and the list goes on and on.

Susie is no different than you or I. We all suffer from a false identity crisis at times. The trick is catching it or reversing it before it destroys you.

I waited for Susie to respond. Her eyes flashed from mine to the floor, then back to me. I could tell she was thinking. What did I mean? Was I going to blame her for her problems? So many people already blamed her and judged her. She couldn't hear it from another doctor. Not me.

But I have to give Susie credit, she pushed all that self-doubt and lies that the world had told her about herself and said, "Yes." I smiled. This was the beginning of her new life. She just couldn't see it yet. I had to reveal the hidden joy that was waiting just around the corner for her.

Sometimes we can't believe our own dreams or new identities. That's why it's important to have someone who can push you in the right direction. Susie was not a weak woman. In fact, she was one of the strongest I have ever had the privilege to help. She had just become disillusioned by her failures and thought these illnesses were all there was to life, that they were what *she* was.

You might be wondering what happened to Susie after our meeting.

"It doesn't take much to make a huge impact on your life."

— Kent MacLeod

We set Susie on a two-month plan. The first month I had her substitute her typical morning breakfast with a high protein smoothie. Every morning, she drank a low carbohydrate smoothie with twenty-five grams of whey protein, fruits, and vegetables.

This was all I had her change in her lifestyle, initially. As you might guess, she was incredulous, but she agreed and stuck to the plan.

One month later, she returned to me. By merely substituting her high sugar intake with a healthy alternative, her blood sugar levels dropped nearly double and she lost fifteen pounds. Most people are unaware of the dangers that high sugar breakfasts have on their health.

Sometimes this is due to ignorance. They just don't know how much sugar is in breakfast foods like cereals or white bread. Needless to say, Susie was ecstatic with the results, but we weren't done yet. I had

Susie continue her smoothie in the mornings but added a customized paleo diet for the rest of her meals.

This consisted primarily of fruits, vegetables, and lean protein. She did this for thirty more days, then came to see me again. Have any ideas of what happened next? If you're thinking, "She reduced her blood sugar levels, eliminated her diabetes, and lost more weight," you'd only be partially right.

Susie's blood sugar levels did drop to normal levels. Her diabetes did disappear. She did lose more weight without doing anything else. She did stop having to take her medication. But there's more. Susie had energy, loads of it!

She was happier. She enjoyed getting out of bed and going out into the world. She no longer hid herself in her home, afraid to venture out. She had a bounce in her step, and coming from a sixty-three-year-old woman, that's a testament in and of itself. She reconnected with friends. She got involved with her community and her family. And people began to notice the life in her.

This all sounds like utopia, but there were struggles along the way. Susie's body went through withdrawal for certain foods and her cravings were relentless. There were times she wanted to quit, she felt so bad. But she was motivated to see results. She wanted her life back.

I remember telling her one day, "I know you're struggling right now, but I cannot hurt you by taking processed foods out of your diet and having you eat as much fruits and vegetables as you want."

Susie is just one of thousands of patients with similar stories that I and my team have been blessed to set free over the years. She, like them, wanted radical change in their lives. But the truth is, it wasn't so much a radical change in diet or lifestyle as it was a mindset shift and believing in her heart that she *could* be more.

Then with a little fine-tuning, that radical change came about. If it only takes a small adjustment to make such grandiose improvements in our well-being and happiness, then why don't more people do it? The reason is *limiting beliefs*.

ALCOHOL, CANNABIS, OPIOIDS, NSAIDS, PPIS, & ANTIBIOTICS

"The struggles with mental illness in our society keep escalating. It's not a coincidence that the problem isn't solved by a pill, anymore that it's a coincidence that this type of illness is worse in those with unhealthy microbiomes."

— Kent MacLeod

The limiting beliefs that govern the modern era of medicine extend beyond mere medicinal benefits. We've narrowed our view with the illusion that drugs heal us. But in fact, they are killing us and forming life-altering habits that leave most of Canada and the United States heavily medicated.

Understanding the effects of each of these seven key culprits to poor or good health is crucial to living an abundant life. Let's dive into each of these in more detail and see how they're impacting our lives and how we can change these.

Our conventional way of thinking:

"The next medication or product will be the one to solve the symptoms of your issue- anxiety, depression, pain, etc."

VS.

A better way to think of it:

"What do I actually need to have a healthy brain?"

We now see that these drugs are not good for brain health and they will not work for long.

What we are ultimately trying to do is to emphasize brain health, not just treat symptoms.

STRESS

While stress may not be seen as a mental disorder, it's quite possibly the most harmful of any factor on the brain and body's well-being. Stress has been linked to heart disease, asthma, obesity, headaches & migraines, fatigue, insomnia, diabetes, anxiety & depression, gastrointestinal problems (IBS, GERD, reflux disease, heartburn), Alzheimer's disease, increased aging, and premature death.

Stress is no joke and must be dealt with to reduce its harmful effects. While it's commonly accepted that the normal way to handle stress is through prescribed antidepressants or seeing a counselor or psychiatrist, it's more difficult for people to believe that balancing their microbiome would improve it, not medication.

Through G.U.T., we can explain to the general population and the medical field that there is a simpler and better way to deal with physical and mental health issues.

According to one study done by the American Nutrition Association, over 70,000,000 people worldwide, every day, suffer from a gastrointestinal (GI) problem. The Journal of Gastroenterology stated that a high percentage of those people going to GI clinics for irritable bowel syndrome also scored high on the anxiety rating scale. There are two primary ways the gut influences anxiety.

The channels are via the vagus nerve and indirect chemical signals.

As we mentioned earlier in the eight gut-brain connections section, the vagus nerve is the direct link from the brain to the gut.

They both are in constant connection and communication with one another. The vagus nerve sends signals and information to and from the brain to the rest of the body. If you're stressed, then more cortisol is pumped into the bloodstream.

In addition to cortisol, this nerve sends hormones, neuropeptides, neurotransmitters, and inflammatory markers like cytokines, and then the immune system signals that something is wrong. And while this stress signal is healthy when you're in a stressful situation and need to take action, it's deadly for the body to maintain that rate of alertness long-term.

I've heard many patients say, "You don't understand the severity of my stress." Whether this is job stress, familial, spousal, financial, sexual, or something else, I've heard just about everything. And I say each time, "I'm not a psychologist. And you're right, I don't understand *your* stress." But what they don't understand, and what I've spent more than thirty-five years testing, researching, and developing, is the direct impact the gut plays on their perception of stress.

When my patients improve their gut health, they report substantial loss of anxiety, despite the fact that nothing else in their life has changed. Meaning, the same stressors that they had initially complained about and blamed for their anxiety and health problems are still present.

As your gut health improves, you become more resilient to stress and illness. We can set out baseline stress by our microbiomes. We emphasize managing our stress, but we never discuss the real change factor: our guts.

ALCOHOLISM

Alcoholism, or alcohol specifically, is the most harmful addiction in Canada and the Unites States (most costly economically and associated with the most deaths statistically). We have all kinds of medications, counseling, Alcoholics Anonymous groups, and more to treat alcoholism. And yet, the problem just keeps getting worse.

Why is that?

Could it be that we aren't addressing the real problem? Could it be that the addiction is not the issue, or the alcohol, but a damaged or compromised microbiome?

I believe so.

We're still using the same drugs to treat alcoholism that we've been using for the last thirty years. The definition of madness is doing the same thing over and over again expecting different results. And while some people succeed in breaking their addiction, most relapse or get worse. Studies have shown that using benfotiamine (a fat-soluble form of vitamin B1) is more effective than these other drugs and harm-reduction therapies.

The methods to treat alcoholism have remained the same, but it's never been approached from the gut. People think that I am crazy when I start talking about nutrition and digestive health in regard to alcoholism, but there is a lot of research emerging to support a microbiome-addiction connection. The microbiome plays an integral role in alcohol addiction and the co-morbidities (side-effects of alcohol abuse, in this case) related to it.

DID YOU KNOW...

The vast majority of patients with alcohol use disorder are vitamin B1, B6, and B12 deficient.

Deficiencies in these three vitamins are associated with nerve damage (neuropathy) and liver failure. Our work has also found that supplementing with these B-vitamins reduces cravings for alcohol more than any other drug. This shouldn't be new to those working within these areas of addiction and treatment, and yet, it might as well be information that is kept top-secret. I've attended multiple conferences where this was never addressed.

Imagine you've suffered from alcoholism for years. You've tried medication, AA groups, counseling, and psychotherapy, but nothing works. In fact, you're worse. You crave the alcohol even more!

Addiction treatment focuses on specific drugs or receptors, but there is no focus on brain health. All alcoholics have disrupted microbiomes, yet we do not target the microbiome at all in alcoholism. You're never going to significantly reduce cravings with these drugs compared to improving microbiome and brain health. And certain vitamins, like vitamin B1, or its fat-soluble form benfotiamine, have shown to be more effective than all of the drugs used for alcoholism.

You may have suffered for years from alcoholism and tried many remedies. Then, by chance, the microbiome is revealed to you and things begin to start making sense. You're taught that by replenishing your gut and nutrient status, you'll recover your health and beat your addiction. You're skeptical at first. Who wouldn't be! Nothing's worked for you, until now.

You adjust your diet according to a gut specialist to kill off the bad bacteria and influencers, and you replenish your body with the good. Within a few short days, you're noticing a positive change. The craving for alcohol is losing its grip on you, and you are feeling better in other ways.

Other health problems are abating. You start sleeping better, your moods have improved, your complexion is brighter, you're smiling more, and you have energy. After you complete your 60-day detox regimen, you don't even want to take a drink.

My claim about the gut as the central factor to poor or thriving health is a bold claim. I know this, but it doesn't mean it's incorrect. In fact, I have the research, studies, evidence, and case studies to prove it. I can't say it often enough: a healthy microbiome is essential to brain health. Conversely, an unhealthy microbiome is associated with mental health issues, addiction, and more serious complications from addiction.

CANNABIS

This topic will bring some controversy. With the legalization of cannabis becoming more and more a hot topic in Canada, the United States, and other countries, it's even more critical to understand the effects this drug can have on the brain and body.

We've already seen how harmful alcohol is on your well-being.

And it's legal!

Since the beginning of time, people have moved from one miracle panacea drug to the next. We're always after that next quick-fix or feel-good-remedy. It's always, "That didn't work, but this will solve all of my problems!"

We see examples of this frame of thinking with the opioid crisis. People are taking opioids and PPIs for pain and digestive problems like they're candy. People rely on antidepressant pills for depression and anxiety without daring to look more deeply into their causes.

I've seen many patients suffering from fibromyalgia and anxiety who use cannabis to manage their symptoms. Every single one of them had altered or deteriorated microbiomes. I'm not against people finding peace and relief from their pain, but I am for making people well instead of merely treating the symptoms. Cannabis is not essential for a healthy brain, but a healthy microbiome is. An inflamed brain will contribute to more pain syndromes, such as fibromyalgia.

Cannabis is a surface/symptomatic solution. It is safer than opioids, and I use it in my practice short-term for pain relief instead of opioids because it has a much safer side-effect profile. For some people, cannabinoids can be very beneficial, but if we truly want to heal, we need to focus on and treat the ultimate underlying cause of a lot of our problems- our microbiomes. I've witnessed hundreds of new medications and drugs being developed that claim to be the "cure-all" only to flop and cause more side effects. I am a proponent of cannabis, but it will not solve all of our health problems.

Cannabinoids are a far better solution to pain than narcotics. If it brings relief, it's better than dealing with pain, anxiety, depression, and any number of health problems. But the ultimate solution is improving our gut health because this will always reduce inflammation and pain.

OPIOIDS

If you're unfamiliar with the term opioids, these are substances that bind with opioid receptors (found in the central & peripheral nervous systems, and the gastrointestinal tract) to treat pain.

However, due to their euphoric effects, many people become dependent on them, abuse them, or use them as recreational drugs. The problem develops as more and higher doses are required to maintain that same effect on pain control.

You may recognize some of the more popular names for the legally prescribed opioids: oxycodone, hydrocodone, codeine, and morphine.

Again, these drugs were created to alleviate pain, but it's only handling the surface problem while disrupting the microbiome through their use. This only leads to a higher likelihood of addiction.

I'd like to offer an alternative way of thinking about pain.

Where did the Opioid Crisis Come From?

For acute pain, opioids are useful, and you can stop using them easily as that acute pain heals, for example, from surgery. But if this pain persists, such as in forms called neuropathic pain, you get inflammation in the nervous system, and this leads to a heightened response to pain. Inflammation of the brain and nervous system can lead to central sensitivity syndrome (CSS). If you give people with this condition opioids, the drugs work short-term, but the actual inflammation does not stop, and can become worse over time.

And giving opioids over time you actually get more pain rather than less. This is called rebound hyperalgesia. You can see why people would keep using more and more opioids in this instance—their pain was not improving. Their doses keep going up and up because of rebound pain. In the past, Big Pharma had taught doctors that for pain syndromes, opioids were not addictive (which was untrue), even though they were not actually treating the pain very well.

A focus on brain health is what is needed to help people's pain. By targeting the microbiome, we can reduce inflammation and calm the nervous system. This is a more effective ultimate treatment for pain and inflammation.

INTERESTING FACT:
CSS is ten times more prevalent in women. And the microbiome has a direct link to estrogen, vitamin B6 & B1 metabolism.

Opioids are meant for short-term pain treatment. However, their highly addictive properties make it hard to stop taking them. There are dangerous side effects from long-term use, such as bone fractures, sleep apnea, respiratory and heart failure, and hyperalgesia (a very painful condition).

So why take opioids in the first place if they have such harmful side effects?

The short answer is because they're easy to administer and they offer immediate relief.

However, just like alcohol, they are addictive and they damage the microbiome, which leads to more serious illnesses and even death. The more imbalanced your microbiome becomes, the more difficult it'll become for you to control your cravings and replace the nutrients that your gut has lost.

If this continues, you'll become more susceptible to something called Leaky Gut Syndrome (LGS). In LGS, the lining of the gastrointestinal tract becomes compromised and toxins from the unhealthy gut can leak into the bloodstream, causing a variety of inflammatory problems throughout the body.

We'll discuss LGS in more detail in Chapter 3 – How to Know When Your Microbiome is Disrupted.

NSAIDS

Nonsteroidal anti-inflammatory drugs (NSAIDs) are a class of drug used to reduce pain, decrease fever, and prevent blood clots. With larger doses, they can potentially minimize inflammation.

Doesn't sound too harmful, does it? In fact, it sounds pretty good. Let's keep reading to see why these drugs aren't all they are hyped up to be and why you should avoid or minimize your intake.

Some popular examples of over-the-counter or prescribed NSAIDs include:

- Aspirin
- Ibuprofen (Advil, Motrin)
- Naproxen (Aleve)
- Celecoxib (Celebrex)

Most degenerative diseases include symptoms of inflammation. Inflammation is associated with all of the following diseases:

- Cancer
- Diabetes
- Coronary Artery Disease
- Alzheimer's disease
- Parkinson's disease
- Heart Attack
- Stroke
- Arthritis

This is a short list of common diseases that affect most of the world's population, primarily in Canada and the United States. I'm willing to make a wager with you. I bet you or someone you know, who suffers or has suffered from one of these terrible diseases, have taken NSAIDs.

The more important question is why. Why does inflammation occur in all of these diseases?

I'm glad you asked. The gut microbiome.

Your gut becomes more permeable (it allows liquids or gases to pass through it) over time, when you repeatedly expose yourself to medications, such as NSAIDs. When your bowels can't process toxins in the body, due to weakness (usually caused by NSAIDs), your body will begin to secrete proteins, bacteria, and other gut-related components into your bloodstream.

This, in turn, results in inflammation. The ironic part of all of this is that the NSAIDs, which you're taking to reduce inflammation, actually cause it. This is just more evidence to show that medication does not cure the problem but instead coats it or causes it to become worse.

Today's research shows a connection between NSAIDs and poor gut health. Through repeated exposure, your gut's ability to act as a barrier between the waste processing system and the body is compromised. And as I stated before, this leads to more inflammation, as well as issues like gluten sensitivity.

Could it be that those allergic to gluten aren't in fact allergic but have damaged or compromised microbiomes? I believe so. As you're beginning to see, all of your health issues come full circle back to the microbiome.

We've been treating our symptoms with no improvement with the WRONG tools! When you address the ACTUAL source, you can cure the REAL problem.

Three issues we face with these drugs are:

1. They are one of the deadliest groups of drugs and very few know of their dangers
2. We know that an unhealthy microbiome can cause inflammation throughout the body and brain
3. These drugs inhibit the production of normal mucosal lining (via inhibition of prostaglandins) and disrupt the microbiome, which can lead to inflammation, ulcers, gastrointestinal bleeds, and leaky gut

If you have lots of inflammation and you use NSAIDs, you may find that you get a much more dramatic improvement in your inflammation once you improve your microbiome compared to using NSAIDs alone. It is also kind of ironic that you take these drugs to reduce inflammation but they can actually cause inflammation.

PPIS (THE QUIET CRISIS)

Proton-Pump Inhibitors (PPIs). These drugs' primary function is to reduce stomach acid production. Suffer from acid reflux or gastrointestinal problems? You've probably been given a PPI to manage your symptoms. In fact, in Canada they are the #3 most prescribed class of drugs. They are given for almost all stomach problems, usually inappropriately, which means that most prescriptions are written in error. This has triggered a quiet crisis, or a "crisis" that no one really knows about. It's a crisis because these drugs damage the microbiome, increasing death rates dramatically in their long-term users. Long-term use of PPIs is now known to be associated with many health problems, such as osteoporosis, dementia, pneumonia, C. Difficile, and kidney failure to mention a few connections.

We keep treating acid as a problem in the stomach, but most of the time, gastrointestinal disease is a problem of a thin mucosal lining of the GI tract. A functional mucosal lining requires a healthy microbiome and can easily handle stomach acid. If you just turn off the acid, the bacteria in your gut shifts toward unhealthy bacteria, which can be a disaster for your microbiome.

One of the easiest things to do for someone's general health is to get them off of their long-term PPI if it is being used inappropriately. NutriChem pharmacists actually sit on the Canadian Deprescribing Committee and one of our major areas of focus is helping patients to come off of inappropriate PPIs.

I know I keep mentioning this, but it bears repeating: your micro-biome is a living organism, which is interconnected with the rest of your body and brain. Just as stress damages and leads to other symptoms or diseases, it also plays an integral part in aggravating your microbiome.

A few PPIs that you might be familiar with or have been prescribed at some point include:

- Omeprazole (Prilosec, Prilosec OTC, Zegerid)
- Lansoprazole (Prevacid)
- Pantoprazole (Pantoloc, Protonix)
- Rabeprazole (Aciphex)
- Esomeprazole (Nexium)
- Dexlansoprazole (Dexilant)

I'm all for bodily relief, but not at the cost of your well-being and microbiome suffering in the long-term. I'd go as far as to say that taking any of these medications is an indicator that your microbiome needs recalibration.

The hardest thing I've learned over the years with the thousands of patients I've helped is their struggle with understanding and knowing the full picture of the gut. Chances are you are not a gastroenterologist, nor do you have any educational or professional training in the area.

This is actually a good thing and a bad thing. It's bad in the sense that you're unaware of the true importance of each of your bodily functions and how to take care of them. It's good because you're starting from square one and can learn afresh, without any preconceived biases.

I'd even wager it's better that you have no prior knowledge; sometimes it's easier to move forward with change when you don't know what to expect. You just know you want to start living the life you were born to enjoy. I'll do my best to explain the gut so you can better understand its importance for your health and why PPIs and other medications are so detrimental to its well-being.

There is a misconception of what the stomach does. Common knowledge might lead one to believe the stomach is where digestion of food and liquid takes place. And while this is partially true (meaning, digestion BEGINS in the stomach), it would be missing the mark.

The acids in the stomach aid in the digestive process. Full digestion really takes place in the small intestine where food and liquid is broken down and absorbed. If you take PPIs, you're altering the pH levels of the stomach acids, which in turn, leads to increased pH (lower acidity) of the small and large intestine, increasing risks for infections.

PPIs dramatically alter the pH of the GI tract, changing all of the bacteria in the small intestine. This can shift the gut towards unhealthy bacteria, such as *C. difficile.*

Maybe you've heard of *E. Coli* and *Salmonella.* But you might not have heard of a more dangerous infection, known as *C. difficile.* The reason why this infection is so dangerous is because it's almost untreatable. Virtually no antibiotic will kill it. And when you increase your PPI intake, you increase your risk of *C. diff* infection.

It's important to note, that your gut normally contains a healthy amount of *C. difficile.* Just as bacteria is necessary for a balanced and healthy gut, so too are "bad" bacteria necessary. The importance is on balance. By maintaining a healthy microbiome, you reduce or completely eliminate your risk of infections and other diseases.

I love analogies. They help take complex ideas and make them easier to understand in everyday terms. And are fun!

I want you to picture your lawn. If you don't own or lease a home, then picture any section of grass, whether at your apartment or even a store. The importance is not the where but that you can see the grass in your mind's eye.

Alright, do you have the grass in sight? Good.

I want you to examine your grass. Is it green? Is it plush? Are there dead spots, weeds, or brown spots? Have insects infested it? Or is your lawn pristine, exuberant, and lush with life? If you're the latter, then you're the envy of all of your neighbors. Don't worry, this analogy is still relevant to you.

See, I told you analogies were fun! Let's keep going.

Take a natural lakeshore. A few items that don't belong in its natural habitat won't damage the entire shoreline. It'll still thrive, and eventually, that which doesn't belong, dies off.

The microbiome behaves the same way. A little good bacteria here and there, some PPIs, NSAIDS, or medications won't hurt the overall stomach microbiome ecosystem, but the more you take them (or allow them to infest your lawn), the quicker the entire lawn (or gut) is destroyed. Pretty soon, your lawn is brown, dead, and lifeless.

Getting your lawn back to life will take some time and effort. It'll require lots of weed killer, pesticide, and fertilizer to shock it back. With the work and the right nutrients, your lawn can recover. That's how you should picture your gut and its effect on the rest of your body.

You may have all of these health problems. It may seem like your entire lawn is infested with insects and weeds and there's no way you'll ever recover. With the right plan and supplements (nutrients), you'll revive your lawn to its full capacity.

Just as weeds can disrupt the ecosystem of your lawn, so too, can PPIs disrupt your microbiome. If you remember nothing else, remember the Grand Unified Theory (G.U.T.), which reminds you to view your body as one vessel with multiple moving parts, and their relationship to every other system of the body, including the brain. Anything you ingest (food, drink, medications, etc.) can affect your microbiome, which in turn, affects the biology of the brain.

I'm encouraged to see modern medicine developing an understanding and awareness of the affects PPIs have on the long-term health of the gut microbiome. Consistent use of PPIs disrupts the gut's ability to absorb key vitamins, minerals, and nutrients, such as calcium, magnesium, iron, vitamin B12 & vitamin C.

Recent studies have now found a direct correlation between long-term use of PPIs and dementia.

If you are taking a PPI medication for uncomplicated heartburn, I would recommend you discuss stopping your PPI with your prescriber as soon as possible!

ANTIBIOTICS

I remember thirty-five years ago when antibiotics were used for just about anything. Colds, bronchitis, mild respiratory issues, you name it. Doctors even prescribed them to children as a preventative, even though there was not a shred of evidence to support that they prevented anything.

The belief at the time was that antibiotics were only good, never harmful. We were wrong.

Yes, they work acutely, when used for the right reasons. However, even one use of antibiotics will disrupt the bacterial structure of your gut microbiome. While antibiotics work to kill off infections, they also kill off the good bacteria that your gut needs to thrive.

The problem comes when people don't replenish the microbiome with probiotics. The more you take antibiotics, the less effective they become, and the more susceptible you become to more harmful infections, like *C. Difficile*.

Eventually, if we continue to overuse them, antibiotics won't work anymore. This is called antibiotic resistance. It's now 2018, and we already have a host of infections that are untreatable by antibiotics. I mentioned C. difficile. There's no good cure, antibiotics are often useless, and it can kill you in the hospital.

There is only one process that has shown promise with combating serious digestive infections like *C. Difficile*. It's known as microbiome stool transplant, or fecal microbiota transplantation. The name is self-explanatory. Your microbiome receives a transplant from a healthy individual's microbiome.

"It's not pretend anymore. We now know that destroying the microbiome has extreme effects on your brain, your immune system, and increases your risk for deadly infections."

— Kent MacLeod

We're finally starting to understand the importance of protecting our gut microbiomes, but we're still a long way away from solving the problem. We now know we can treat a surplus of conditions by reviving the microbiome. And yet, we're still consuming these harmful substances and wonder why we feel so bad and why so many people are sick or dying.

The conversation needs to change.

The days of viewing antibiotics as the simple, go-to solution for our illnesses is no more. There will be resistance from pharmaceutical companies, but the best way to prevent something from being mass produced is not to buy it.

Think about how much antibiotics you've been consuming through the groceries you buy, without even realizing it. What do you think most of the meat you eat has in it? Most farmers use antibiotics on those animals. It's vital that you ensure what you are consuming was not grown or raised with antibiotics, pesticides, or non-natural ingredients.

It'll cost more at first, but eventually, the industries will adapt to us.

BRAIN POWER TIP

In our busy world, with so many options presented to us every second, it's easy to become overwhelmed. We've grown accustomed to quick-fixes or easy solutions. We're conditioned to seek the "best deals" and latch onto immediate gratification and pleasure.

You have a headache? Take this.
Your stomach hurts? Here, take this pill.
You have chronic panic attacks and anxiety? Take two of these, three times a day. You'll feel better.

The next time you're presented with "Take this pill" to fix your health problems, stop. I want you to do a self-reflection of your life. If you've been taking medication for years and have only seen your health get worse, then you have your answer.

If you've never taken medication, but are tempted to start, approach with caution. Learn from those around you who have suffered as a result to these supposed "safe" options and "quick-fixes". Your health and life mean more than that.

Wouldn't it be nice to find an alternative that doesn't result in you needing to take more medication, for the rest of your life, and that doesn't cause more illness?

If there were a way you could feel better in just a week's time, or that would reduce your health problems by 70%, in just thirty days, would you try it?

This may sound like science fiction because you've become disillusioned by modern medicine and its assurances that it knows what it's doing. But I can assure you, through the thousands of people I've helped, and the millions of hours that went into this research, that a cure is possible, and it doesn't require another pill.

Want to test my theory?

For the next week, just one week, I want you to eat only healthy, natural foods. These include fruits, vegetables, and high protein sources (only organic). I'd encourage you to use an organic whey protein mix instead of meat if you're unsure whether it's been injected with antibiotics.

Healthy foods generate a balanced microbiome. Wouldn't you want something that eliminates your health problems, instead of just covers them up for a little while?

It's only a week. Give it a shot and see if I'm lying. I guarantee it'll change your life.

"It is in your moments of decision that your destiny is shaped."

— Tony Robbins, #1 NYT bestselling author of Unlimited Power and Awaken the Giant Within, life coach, and philanthropist

CHAPTER 3

HOW TO KNOW WHEN YOUR MICROBIOME IS DISRUPTED

"The human body is filled with triggers and alerts that let you know when it is not functioning properly. Only the individual experiencing the disruption can initiate discovering the reasons for the change."

— Kent MacLeod

The gut microbiome is a complex, living organism. As we've discussed, it is multilayered and comprised of numerous moving parts that interact with different parts of the body. When one section malfunctions, the rest of the body performs at a reduced efficiency. But unlike injuries like a broken leg or a cut, the microbiome's dilemma is more complicated and life-altering.

I say this not to allude to it being some mystical entity that you'll never understand. On the contrary, the microbiome is complex in that it's interlinked with multiple layers and facets of the human body, both physical and psychological.

When we understand the channels through which the gut microbiome operates, we can monitor those corridors for any adverse changes, blockages, or disruptions. But how do you know when your microbiome has suffered a catastrophic failure or interference?

Awareness.

Socrates said it best when he penned, *"The unexamined life is not worth living."* Without self-examination, we're living blindly. And without action on that awareness, we're living foolishly.

"When I discover who I am, I'll be free."

— Ralph Ellison

These days, we hear a lot about self-reflection, meditation, self-awareness, and self-enlightenment. Every day, we're encouraged to look inward and be our own boss, to control our own destiny, and to manifest our inner worlds in our lives. Yet a lot of this is directed at mental states, ignoring our physical health. In the midst of all of this good inward examining, we can overlook matters that surreptitiously dictate our well-being and quality of life.

We've been discussing the primary functions of the microbiome and how internal and external forces can disrupt it. We briefly touched on two critical conditions that lead to an increased release of toxins in the bloodstream and negatively impact the body as a whole, as well as the microbiome.

These two conditions are the leaky gut and inflammation. We'll break each one down so you can fully understand the cause of each, how they affect your body and mind, and how to stop or prevent these conditions from occurring.

Have you ever had someone tell you, "You should stop being so negative," "Just do the right thing," or, some other prescriptive trope meant well. Or maybe you've told yourself something like this before. Perhaps you're always sick and never have energy to engage with the world around you, and as a result, you've become critical and negative.

Maybe this has pushed your friends and family away. Maybe you did it by choice. No matter the situation or the reason, it's never quite as simple as saying, "Just change your mind," or "Do the right thing." Of course, you'd like to! You don't want to stay sick for the rest of your life. You're tired of feeling miserable and being alone.

But being aware—the essential first step—is only part of the solution. the next crucial step is to know *what to do* and *how*. In this chapter, I'll show you how you can harness your awareness of these harmful conditions to affect positive change, righting those imbalances.

How? By teaching you how to listen to your body.

LEAKY GUT — THE INVISIBLE DESTROYER OF WORLDS (AKA YOUR HEALTH)

The term "leaky gut" is not a scientific or official medical term. It's a phrase commonly used to describe a severe condition in the gut microbiome where the intestinal lining has become compromised. This breach in the intestinal lining is usually caused by the lack of essential nutrients in your diet.

Even more commonly, leaky gut is a direct result of your diet, environment, culture, stress, drug and medication intake. Leaky gut primarily affects people in developed nations. Impoverished nations have their own share of troubles with the gut, but we'll touch base on that a little later.

I'd like to pause here for a moment to clear up any misconceptions you may have about the gut. Before I went to pharmaceutical school some thirty-five years ago and learned about the gut microbiome, I thought of the gut as just the stomach. An organ just like any other in the body that digested or stored food. Perhaps you think the same.

While this is not acutely inaccurate, it's not the whole truth. If you've ever been to court, you may recall being sworn in. A common phrase you'll be asked to repeat is "the whole truth," entailing that there is a difference between the truth and the whole truth.

Sometimes the whole truth is not required to help someone or to achieve a certain outcome. "Did you take out the trash?" your wife might ask. You think, "Yikes! I forgot to but I'll do it right now" so you say, "Yes, dear," then go take out the trash. Or, you get the dreaded question, "Does this dress make me look fat?"

If you're posed this question, just smile, and say you look beautiful and move on before you're ensnared in a trap. Naturally, I'm teasing but it's for good reason. Truth and the whole truth are not synonymous, just as the gut is not the same as the stomach or just an organ. There's more to everything than what might meet the eye.

I want to challenge you to join me on a path of discovery, to see your gut as more than just another organ that tells you when you're hungry or sick, but something much more amazing. Pretend you're standing in front of a waterfall. The mountain soars a thousand feet up and disappears into the clouds. The water cascades and hammers into the rocks below. You're off to the side and watch as it merges with the river and flows away.

It's beautiful, isn't it? You could stand there all day listening to that sound. But we're not here to enjoy the scenery or listen to the melodious music of nature, we want to dive deeper. Step up to the waterfall and stretch your hand through it. See how your hand goes right through? Now step through with your entire body.

If you did, you're probably soaking wet—in our imaginary example— and are now standing on the other side of the water. Maybe it's a cave or just a small inlet underneath the mountain. Either way, the waterfall acted as a thin barrier between where you were and where you are now.

The gut microbiome is the same—metaphorically. The microbiome is your barrier between health and sickness. It's directly connected with your brain and the rest of your body. Much like the waterfall flows from the mountaintop to the valley below, your gut uses tools to connect to your body. We talked about these in more depth in the chapter before.

Now let's go one step further. When your gut is compromised, the toxins cannot be contained as they should. If the river somewhere on the mountain or in the valley were to be blocked by fallen rocks or trees, the flow would stop and the water would become stagnant and full of harmful bacteria. You would not want to drink from that pool of water.

A similar thing occurs with your gut. When your gut is disrupted, the thin barrier can no longer contain the harmful toxins that it prevents from spreading to the body, and those same toxins are now penetrating through and into the bloodstream through the gut's permeable membrane. As a result, the rest of your body and brain become susceptible to viruses, infections, inflammation, and diseases.

Some of the most common problems that result from leaky gut, are the following:

- Irritable Bowel Syndrome (IBS) — Roughly 25-45 million people in the United States suffer from this condition, and two out of three are female.
- Chronic depression and/or anxiety — The World Health Organization (WHO) estimates that roughly 350 million people, worldwide suffer from depression and/or anxiety.

(This number climbs every year.)

- Autoimmune diseases or disorders (Rheumatoid Arthritis, Crohn's Disease)
- Ulcerative Colitis (causes inflammation in the digestive tract)
- Chronic Fatigue Syndrome
- Liver disease (more prevalent in alcohol addictions)
- Diabetes Type 1 & 2

These diseases or disorders are not all-inclusive. If you have a leaky gut, you may suffer from low energy, cognitive impairments (memory loss, anxiety, lack of concentration), nutritional deficiencies, further digestive disruptions or complications, and you may even develop food allergies.

If you experience any of these symptoms (and chances are, you do), you need to take immediate action on recovering your microbiome's balance. Just a small "leak" can cause serious damage to your well-being and health.

I don't say this to scare you, unless it prompts you to take action. The microbiome is not something to play games with. It's the source of your health or its deterioration. A quote by Hippocrates, used at the beginning of Chapter 1 states, "All disease starts in the gut." Even he, some twenty-four hundred years ago, knew the "whole truth" about the human body.

As humans, we're blinded by the illusion that progression is made from age to age, that things from the past can't possibly be as sophisticated as what we come up with today. We think that just because modern medicine has evolved from previous centuries' procedures or methods, that it's better. Yes, we have made significant leaps in the medicinal and technological realms, but not as much as you might think. The same medicine we created to cure illness also creates it.

Here's some science for you.

Leaky gut is caused by compromised tight junctions between cells. Normally, enterocytes allow good nutrients to pass through while blocking the entry of pathogens (things that cause diseases) into the bloodstream.

It's when these single cells and the tight junction connections between them are compromised that the problem begins.

You might have already assumed by our explanation of the gut that everything is connected. But there's always a gap. I'll give you an example. Hold your hands in the air, with your fingers secured together. No matter how hard you try to close your fingers, there will always be a gap between them. The same occurs if you place both hands together, palm-to-palm.

This image serves only to depict what happens on a molecular level. There is space between every cell in our bodies. This space for an enterocyte is called a tight junction. These tight junctions are produced by enterocytes that rely on energy from gut bacteria, and these gut bacteria use fibers to live and to produce energy. The best way to imagine these tight junctions is like tiny molecular doors between the intestines and the bloodstream. On one side of the door are the intestines. On the other, the bloodstream. When your body's nutritional level is depleted or compromised, this "door" doesn't function properly.

If your bedroom were full of water and the only thing keeping it from flooding your house was the door, wouldn't you want to ensure that door was stable, strong, and secure? What would happen if your bedroom door was cracked open? What if it were wide open?

So, what causes your "doorway" to become cracked or wide open?
- Lack of soluble fiber (prebiotics): Your gut bacteria need this fiber to fuel the enterocytes to actually build tight junctions and maintain the gastrointestinal lining.
- Poor diet: E.g. standard North American Diet of high sugar, processed foods, low vegetable intake.
- Lack of exercise: Exercise is a necessary physiological stressor to promote a healthy gut.
- Psychological stress: We've already touched on how detrimental stress is for the microbiome. Stress produces cortisol, and excess cortisol damages the gastrointestinal lining

- Bacteria in the gut: Do you have more bad than good?
- Medications or drugs: Are you taking over-the-counter medications daily? What about prescribed or illegal? Many of these harm the gut's ecosystem.
- Alcohol consumption: unhealthy, copious amounts of alcohol wreak havoc on the microbiome
- Inflammation (the big killer) is believed to be the root cause of many diseases

Picture your microbiome as a space suit. It's the only thing keeping you alive in space. If it gets cracks, you lose oxygen. If the sunshield malfunctions, you get blinded by the sun. If any part of the suit fails to work or gets damaged, you're in for trouble. The actual energy for the space suit is soluble fiber! Your spacesuit battery relies on fiber to run! The microbiome is the motor for the suit, and fibers are the fuel.

Your microbiome does not discriminate. It responds to what is *in* it. You want to make sure it's responding to the things that encourage good health. When your gut is damaged, harmful substances leak into your bloodstream.

Usually, this is fine because the immune system kicks in and attacks the bad stuff. However, when you have a leaky gut, your immune system stays active too long and then can no longer differentiate between good and bad substances. This in turn enables these harmful substances to flow through your bloodstream to the rest of the body.

And before you know it, you're suffering from chronic illnesses like inflammation and digestive disruptions. The only way to recover from these ailments is by healing the gut microbiome. Medications only deal with the surface problems, meanwhile, the root problem is worsening and causing more "cracks" in the body and brain.

INFLAMMATION — THAT NASTY BUGGER!

This is quite possibly the biggest culprit for major diseases and conditions. Inflammation can occur when foreign substances are released into the bloodstream, such as through a leaky gut.

However, inflammation gets a bad name. It's actually a good thing. The problem comes when it's chronic and uncontrolled.

> **INTERESTING FACT:**
> Inflammation is the body's natural defense mechanism to heal damaged cells or attack foreign pathogens and is part of the body's immune response. Without it, we could not heal from infections, damaged tissues, or simple wounds. However, when inflammation becomes constant and excessive, many medical conditions can arise.

Have you ever heard the phrase, "Everything in moderation"? It holds true here. Too much inflammation leads to more serious health concerns, like cancer or rheumatoid arthritis.

Picture it this way: the opposite of brain health is brain inflammation.

The G.U.T. Theory dictates that brain inflammation is intimately connected to the gut. Brain inflammation is very often caused by gut inflammation. Many diseases involving the brain have one primary factor in common: brain inflammation. Included here are Parkinson's disease, addictions, depression, anxiety, traumatic brain injury, autism, ADHD, dementia, and brain fog. And when inflammation from the gut spreads to the brain, it leads to many mental health conditions. You could argue that virtually all mental illness has brain inflammation as a root cause.

If the gut is inflamed, that inflammation spreads to the entire body. Inflammatory substances, such as cytokines, can spread from an inflamed gut into the bloodstream and into joints, muscles, the brain, nervous system (e.g. in fibromyalgia), and organs. When you improve gut inflammation, you mitigate inflammation throughout the entire body, including brain inflammation, nervous system inflammation, and joint inflammation.

Those who suffer from diabetes, chronic renal failure, vitamin B deficiency, under-active thyroid, or alcoholism should pay close attention to nervous system inflammation.

Throughout this book, I share stories and testimonials from patients I have helped to restore their microbiomes and eliminate their health problems. However, with all of my instructing and coaching on the subject, I failed to incorporate this self-diagnosis into my own life.

I never believed it mattered to me because I was mindful of my diet, my exercise, my stress levels—you know, the signs I told you to watch out for. This serves to reinforce what I said at the start of this chapter, *it's not the awareness, but the action that matters.*

For most of my life, I played competitive tennis. And as my body aged, my ego and competitiveness didn't. I never backed down from a match, even if the opponent was half my age. The problem was never the opponent, but the after-effects of such a grueling match.

My knees would ache for days. I'd be benched from playing tennis for a week and was forced to bike just to loosen up my joints. Typical "old guy syndrome"? I thought so too. The common misnomer is that inflammation only happens to old people or those who are out of shape. I was neither. Well, age is just a number, right?

Fortunately, I came to my senses and decided to test myself like I do my patients. As it turned out, my microbiome wasn't as healthy as I thought, even with my fairly healthy lifestyle. I assigned myself to a microbiome reboot, or gut makeover. I like those makeover shows, don't you!

I won't lie. When I tell my patients the first few days or week will be rough, as their bodies adjust, it sounds easy. It's anything but! I felt like I was dying! And I wasn't even in that bad of shape (health wise). I was starving all of the time.

I carried a bag of organic apples everywhere I went. I was munching down on those things like they were candy. I consumed thousands of calories every day just from apples. During my microbiome makeover, I single-handedly kept the apple industry in business.

There is a positive to all of this though. While my body rebooted itself, I lost weight. Even though I consumed more fruits and vegetables than I had in my entire life, I was still losing weight. Weight loss is not as simple as calories in and out as I was taught when I was young. I believe that your body weight set point is dictated by your microbiome, not just calories in and out. This weight loss reminded me that my microbiome was shifting in the right direction. In the first days of "detox," you do feel hungry. As I tell my patients, "You're starving out the bad stuff." Often, when people are addicted to certain foods, I know I am not speaking to that person's mind, I am speaking to their unhealthy gut bacteria that crave certain foods required for their survival.

By the end of my 30-day microbiome reboot, my inflammation had reduced by 90%. I returned to my "youthful" self and the days when I would play competitive tennis. I had more energy, no soreness, and no inflammation.

This got me to thinking like so many of my patients, "Why didn't I do this sooner?!" It's funny how life can twist you up. You may *know* all of the knowledge in the universe, but wisdom is knowing what to *do* with it. This microbiome shift can be really difficult because your gut bacteria dictates your brain's cravings and behavior. It is not as simple as mind over body. It is microbiome over brain. It is like treating any addiction, rooted in chemistry. Your gut keeps you eating junk food even though you know it is junk! Your bad bacteria in the microbiome hijacks your brain's reward systems! Ever since my revival, as I like to call it, I've been able to help even more patients have their own breakthroughs.

The microbiome helps with more than just our health; greater health means greater performance overall. I learned this firsthand even though I had been helping thousands of people for years. The answer to my inflammation was right before my eyes, or in this case, in my gut.

Improving something like inflammation is what I like to call "kill-off" effects, through the proper diet. As you starve out the bad, you promote growth for the good bacteria to thrive. This experience opened my eyes to a larger principle.

Before you judge someone, you must first put yourself in their shoes, as the saying goes. In the case of health professionals, it's crucial we live what we preach. We must do this not only to lead by example, but to continue our own self-development and awareness. Sometimes even coaches need reminding and a boost of encouragement.

Consider how many of us think that overweight people have willpower issues, that their mental health is somehow tied up in their inability to stay away from junk food. I know I've judged people that way and you probably have too. But what if it's not a willpower issue? What if those people simply have severely disrupted microbiomes? Overweight people are blamed for not being mentally strong enough to tackle their addictions when their body is playing an unfair trick on them and telling the brain to feed them junk or else.

It's humbling to try to take one's own medicine. And enlightening. My self-experiment taught me that without the microbiome model, we can't treat people properly and will only continue to burden them with the stigma that they can't harness the willpower to change. Fortunately, thanks to the G.U.T. theory, we don't have to do that anymore.

BRAIN POWER TIP

If this chapter hit a nerve with you—pun intended—I'd encourage you to do a full self-assessment of your lifestyle, your diet, and life choices. Even a little tweaking can have huge results.

As I tell my patients, "If this one shift in your diet improved your health by 70% or more, or better yet, eliminated it entirely, would you do it?"

The answer is always yes, but the real issue comes with follow-through. I believe in you. You can finally live the life you were called to and stop living in fear, anxiety, or pain. It all starts with recalibrating your microbiome. And it might be as simple as adjusting what you're eating for thirty days.

I want to extend a challenge to you. It's the same one I give to all of my patients and to myself. It's a simple, yet profound shift to correcting your microbiome. Are you ready?

For the next 30 days, I want you to incorporate the following prebiotic-rich foods into your diet. I'm not even asking you to change anything else, just add these to what you eat every day. Prebiotics induce growth and activity of beneficial microorganisms in your gut.

You may already eat some of these. If so, keep doing it and eat more! I'll also note, buy organic to ensure your food was not treated or grown with antibiotics or pesticides (two destroyers of gut microbiomes).

- asparagus
- chicory root
- dandelion greens (If only you had known these were healthy as a kid. Now you can tell your parents *I told you so!*)
- garlic
- Jerusalem artichokes
- leeks
- onion
- cold potatoes (cooled potato starch is a prebiotic)

Do this and I guarantee you'll see an improvement in your microbiome and your health.

"Every day brings new choices."

— Martha Beck

Disclaimer: Everyone's body is different, and proper absorption can be a problem with some of the foods on this list. Low FODMAP diet patients must be cautious of certain vegetables, such as garlic and onions.

CHAPTER 4

RESPECT THE MICROBIOME

"One of the greatest disservices you can do for your health and well-being is to discredit options that don't follow the big pharmacy line-of-reasoning. The sources of healing that your body requires can come from the earth."

— Kent MacLeod

We've discussed what the gut microbiome is and how it positively or negatively affects your body and mind. We've also touched on the top influences that damage your microbiome and what that disruption can lead to.

In this chapter, we'll dive in on what a full-body assessment might look like if you were to come to our clinic in Ottawa. And since not everyone will be able to visit us in-person, I want to shed some light on that process, what it looks like, and what the outcome usually consists of. We regularly assess and work with patients from all over the world via correspondence.

At NutriChem, it's all about solving the root issue in someone's life. We bypass the surface-level ailments and symptoms to pinpoint the main culprit to poor health. Our guiding question with every client is "What is causing this person distress in their body?"

Awareness of what is happening to you is one thing. It allows us to know there is a problem. But in order to remedy that and drastically improve your health, we must navigate and understand the why. Why is it happening? Or what is causing it?

Whether you suffer from digestive issues, inflammation, hormonal imbalances, depression, anxiety, or some other debilitating or psycho-logical-altering symptom, there is always an underlying reason. Our goal is to find out what that is and then make things right. Our motto, after all, is "Root. Restore. Recalibrate."

I believe there are four distinct questions you should be thinking about before you visit us at NutriChem or another clinic that specializes in gut therapy.

1. What's your goal (or desired outcome) for visiting the facility?
2. What can you expect during your visit?
3. What's involved during your full-body screening process?
4. What happens after the testing concludes?

These four areas are just the tip of the iceberg.

Our treatment model is best demonstrated in this health pyramid:

Symptom
management

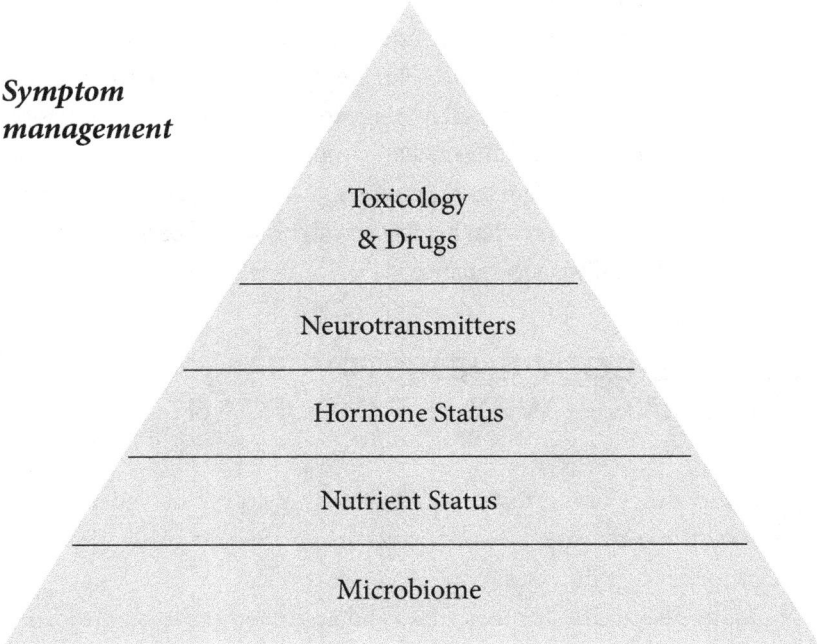

Toxicology
& Drugs

Neurotransmitters

Hormone Status

Nutrient Status

Microbiome

Root Cause

"The best conversations for real solutions begin with understanding your baseline for all your nutrients, hormones, and within the microbiome."

— Kent MacLeod, founder of NutriChem

In the last three decades, I've been fortunate to witness incredible life transformations with my clients. I've had clients on their death beds or on the verge of complete psychological collapse return to full life, energy, and a new revival in their bodies and minds.

I'm eternally indebted to these people. They were brave to seek help and to stick to the process. They allowed me to use my expertise and passion to cure their microbiomes and radically improve their lives. There is no better experience in life than to help someone achieve their goals and find healing. Seeing so many go from helplessness to joy and hope is astounding!

They each finally got the chance to live the life they were meant to live.

THE FULL-BODY CHEMISTRY SCREENING — WHY IT'S IMPORTANT

People are weary about tests. We've grown up to picture hospitals or clinics as these disease-infested areas where people go to die or be treated for serious illnesses.

Many people are sick these days and aren't getting any better. They take the medications their doctors prescribe and follow regimens but nothing helps. They grow sicker by the second with no end in sight. I've seen it too many times to look away. My life has been devoted to creating a successful and sensible alternative that holds real promise for people.

As I've said before, despite the devastating real truth about *modern* medicine, most doctors do want to help their patients get well or find a cure. They are simply ill-equipped to effectively help someone. It all comes down to knowing where to look, then having the tools and resources to do something about the problem.

If you're someone struggling with chronic illnesses or find you aren't performing optimally, you'll benefit from a body chemistry screening.

What is the Full-body Chemistry Screening?
We call it the **Body Chemistry Balancing (BCB) Test** at NutriChem.

Except when patients come in suffering from an acute cold or allergy, the full-body chemistry screening analyzes their body's ecosystems to determine where the problems might originate and how to correct them. This unique test supplies us with the vital information on your chemical composition and helps us learn if there are any molecular inconsistencies.

If there are, we pinpoint these for further analysis to lock in the root cause of your health abnormalities. Over the last thirty years, the majority of my patients' diagnoses came down to a disparaged microbiome, which further impacted their brains.

While there are thousands of symptoms, I've seen eight primary ones that patients suffer from. These include:
- anxiety
- depression
- irritability
- fatigue
- chronic infections
- infertility
- inflammation
- drug and alcohol abuse or addictions

Every single one of these can be improved by around 70% or completely wiped out after one 30-day plan. This is our specialty at NutriChem.

The Body Chemistry Balancing Test begins with a urine and blood sample. I told you it wasn't so bad. If you're someone who's averse to needles or blood work, don't worry. This isn't like the cupping or bloodletting that physicians performed on sick patients for nearly two thousand years. We only need a little. You can keep the rest of your blood.

These two preliminary tests check the following key markers in the body.
- **Microbiome Assessment Panel** — our main lab assessment tool
- **Stool Test** – reveals the levels of distinct strains of bacteria

in the gastrointestinal tract and any other issues that would cause problems for the microbiome.

- **Organic acids**
- **Dietary and symptom analysis**

Other Tests:

- **Antioxidant Panel** — Antioxidants protect your cells from free radicals (molecules produced by food digestion or exposure to harmful substances like tobacco smoke or radiation).
- **Hormone Panel** — Men and women are alike in that hormones are directly linked to many problems or conditions, both in the gut and the brain. It's vital to assess the levels of testosterone, estrogen, progesterone, and growth hormones in the patient's bloodstream.
- **Vitamin D (& Other Vitamins and Minerals e.g. Calcium)**— Not enough vitamin D in your bloodstream can result in several harmful diseases. Vitamin D partners with calcium to build and maintain your bones. It also reduces your risk of developing cancer, cardiovascular diseases, diabetes, and bacterial or viral infections.
- **Neurotransmitter Function** — We assess the proper firing (function) of both excitatory and inhibitory neurotransmitters. Improper neurotransmitter activity will hinder the brain's ability to communicate with the body and send the correct signals, responses, or instructions.
- **Metabolism Panel** — This allows us to see how the body is producing energy from food, determine the health of the kidneys, and measure blood sugar levels, and electrolytes. This panel looks at the following elements:
- *Calcium* — Enables cells to function properly.
- *Carbon dioxide* — Measures how the kidneys and lungs are functioning.
- *Chloride* — Affects the body's management of fluids.

- *Creatinine* — Marker of kidney function.
- *Glucose* (blood sugar) — Source of your body's energy.
- *Potassium* — Vital to cell health.
- *Sodium* — Ensures that cells, tissues, and blood receive the appropriate supply of water.
- *Urea nitrogen* — By-product of a healthy kidney.
- **Energy Production Panel** — Demonstrates how well your body produces energy based on your nutrient and mineral levels.
- **Mineral & Vitamin Deficiencies** — Assesses the levels of minerals and vitamins in the bloodstream. Imbalances lead to poor body function.
- **Blood Count** — Measures the count of red blood cells, white blood cells, hemoglobin (proteins in red blood cells that carry oxygen), hematocrit (proportion of red blood cells to plasma in the blood), and platelets (instrumental in blood clotting).
- **Genetic Testing** — Perform a gene analysis for drug and nutrient metabolism.

In addition to these panels, the Body Chemistry Balancing Test provides information regarding nutrients, mitochondrial status, detoxification pathways (and their nutritional statuses), thyroid function, adrenal function, and more.

This compiled assessment represents your body's chemical makeup. We use these results to paint the picture of what's occurring inside your gut, body, and brain. We begin with the microbiome, as all fruit (outcomes) stems from it.

"An imbalanced microbiome can impact other areas of your body, just as problems in other areas of your body can impact your microbiome. The body—as a full unit—is meant to work in support of its best overall health."

— Kent MacLeod

Through this precise full-body screening we're able to leverage those results to provide a solution and plan-of-attack to enable rapid relief, and a lessening or complete eradication of symptoms.

The important aspects to take away from this section is not what everything means, but to know they all play an integral part in your microbiome's health. These results are for your personal clinician who will take this information and formulate your unique plan.

YOUR PLAN OF ATTACK — WHAT TO DO NEXT

"To keep the body in good health is a duty...otherwise, we shall not be able to keep our mind strong and clear."

— Buddha

You've completed your Body Chemistry Balancing Test and your clinician has reviewed your results with you. Now what?

Have you ever tried a diet only to give up or not find lasting results? What about those infomercials that promise flat abs, wrinkle-free skin, and good health? If you've tried any of these, which I'm sure many of you have, you've most likely become disillusioned by the whole idea of diet and exercise, or good health for that matter.

It all seems like some mystical fairy garden in an imaginary world only for a select few unicorns, but not you. I'm here to tell you this fantasy exists and can be your reality without selling your kidneys on the black market.

All you need is a reboot. Even computers need to be refreshed from time-to-time to install updates or clear out the cache. A 30-day reboot is all you need to restart your system. If I said you'd reduce or completely eliminate your health problems in just thirty days, would you do what I told you?

For many people, their problems can be improved through a simple 30-day body reboot. These usually start with an honest conversation about your current lifestyle, diet (what you eat), allergies/sensitivities, medical conditions, and any prescribed or over-the-counter (OTC) medications you're taking (including any illicit drugs).

You may be disenfranchised with the term diet, but that's all your body needs. A diet is merely what you put into your body. It's not restrictive, it's selective. Your personal clinician creates a unique diet plan for you to initiate and maintain for thirty days. For those requiring an additional boost to kick-start their recovery, a combination of multivitamins and supplements are incorporated into your plan.

NutriChem does not endorse a one-size-fits-all approach to microbiome stimulation and recovery. We tailor every plan precisely to the patient's needs, based on their Body Chemistry Balancing Test results. That's why all of those fancy diets or exercises don't work for you. Every person's body is unique and responds differently to external stimuli. The key is in knowing how it works and then implementing a precise plan to work with the natural flow, not against it.

This is a revolutionary approach to medicine and treatment, as opposed to the pharmaceutical industry's solution: just medicate with the same drug. Rinse. Repeat.

We live by a different code.

Personalized Health Solutions, as our tagline suggests, are all about individual treatment plans. **We practice what is known as** precision medicine. Just as no two fingerprints are the same, no two people require the same treatment. We don't believe in running tests, reviewing, supplying a plan, then letting people go away on their own.

We pair every patient with a nutritionist to guide them on their unique and personalized nutrition program. In addition, if medication, addiction, or abuse is a playing factor, we also incorporate a "deprescribing" program to help wean you off drugs without crazy side effects and painful withdrawals.

AN ALTERNATIVE TO THE BODY CHEMISTRY BALANCING TEST SCREENING

Not everyone will require the full scope of the Body Chemistry Balancing Test screening. Oftentimes, individuals are only searching for a simple solution to feeling better.

For those individuals, we offer a tailored but less intensive approach. People find that this alternative works for those patients that fall within a specific set of parameters. Usually, they have one or more of the following indicators:

- Take several different medications
- Suffer from mental health problems
- Suffer from digestive problems (linked to mental disorders)
- Suffer from fatigue (low energy levels)
- Suffer from pain
- Suffer from addiction

They often share the same viewpoint: "Nothing is working! I take all of these pills and I feel worse, not better."

When I sit down with these people and review their medical history and health problems, I often discover that no one has ever talked to them about their microbiome or approached their health issues from that vantage point. While I am not surprised by this, it disheartens me that so many people suffer needlessly when a simple, yet profound solution is readily available, with minimal side effects and a positive outcome. All that is required is a change in perspective and food choices.

I cannot emphasize enough that modern medicine is flawed. The evidence that the gut and brain are interconnected is overwhelming, and even those that are aware of this link are still ill-equipped to apply it to real patients.

The Biology of the Brain is simply the concept that brain health is determined by gut health. If you want to change how your brain functions, you can. Whether it's a negative or positive result is up to the method you prescribe to. Would you rather continue to take medications you can barely pronounce that continue to manage the symptoms of brain inflammation, or try proven natural products and foods that are essential for brain health? Why not follow a proven, natural remedy that has lasting results, doesn't require constant treatment, and results in no harmful side effects?

You can achieve the desired end with natural ingredients.

Those with mental disorders may be concerned that they will still need to see a psychiatrist, psychologist, or counselor for healing. Sometimes, this is the case, but I've personally witnessed thousands who no longer need those specialists once they address their gut microbiome and begin the healing process.

I'm a supporter of counseling. I believe many people should seek professional help for mental health disorders or to work through difficult life experiences, but it's not an absolute requirement for a healthy, functioning mind, body, and soul. Science has shown evidence of the reverse— for example, digestive issues are responsible for and related to anxiety in as much as 90% of cases.

I understand what I'm saying is hard to accept. It may sound foolish or crazy. It sounds crazy because we think that our brain is separate from the rest of our bodies. But every new invention or breakthrough in mankind's history has come through thinking beyond present limits. Bravery is vital for new approaches to take hold. If you're like me and keep up with the burden of proof, you don't feel crazy, you feel enlightened.

With several thousand patients now living healthy, full lives since I began this over thirty years ago, don't take my word for it, take theirs. You can read through the many testimonials of people just like you who have gone through a short, 30-day reboot and now have lasting, radical results. Have a look at Chapter 12 — Find Your Success Like They Did!

We follow proven, scientific truths about our bodies, our minds, and the world around us. The 30-day reboot focuses on clearing out the gunk in your gut. We follow this up by supplying the newly revived microbiome with power (probiotics and prebiotics).

At this point, it's no longer a restricted diet. In fact, that would be harmful to the microbiome. We emphasize and teach a balanced, holistic approach to eating. Now that we've flushed out your microbiome and resurrected it, there's no need to heavily restrict what you eat, only maintain and listen to your body.

We break this down in more detail in Chapter 7 — Diet.

At the end of the day, NutriChem believes in one thing: empowering people to live better, more fulfilling lives. Wouldn't it be incredible if you no longer…

… suffered from chronic health problems?

… had to take boodles of expensive medication only to "treat" symptoms of the problem (Think of all the money you'd be saving!)

… were required to adhere to some overly strict diet or regimen to maintain a healthy lifestyle or see life-long and permanent improvements?

…were confined by limited science and only had to incorporate natural ingredients (fiber, probiotics, custom-blended supplements) to manage a balanced and effective microbiome?

...were in a constant state of "treatment" but were actually healed from all of your health problems or disorders?

...had to suffer through life but could finally *LIVE* life the way you want and were meant to?

Life-change doesn't need to be expensive, time-consuming, or difficult. It's simple. There's a reason why thousands fly across the globe to visit us at our facility in Ottawa, Canada. They're catching on to the truth of an unparalleled breakthrough that the majority are unaware even exists.

Now you're in the .001%. What will you do with the knowledge you now have? Take control of your life by addressing your microbiome before it's too late.

I'll share more about this process in greater detail in Chapters 7-10, which cover Microbiome Mapping.

BRAIN POWER TIP

I've shared a lot of information up to this point. It's time for you to take a break and step away from the book. Let this knowledge settle in. As you do, perform a simple, self-assessment of your current health. Be honest with yourself and use your perspective, not someone else's, not even mine.

Ask yourself the following probing questions. Remember, be brutally honest! Only you will know the truth...

- Do I take prescription medication for a chronic condition that is not improving?
- Do I take over-the-counter (OTC) medication for any of these chronic conditions?
- Do I use drugs or alcohol in excess?
- Have my prescribed or OTC medications caused other side effects or health problems that require me to take more medication?
- Is my digestive system easily upset or problematic (e.g. frequent gas, bloating, constipation or diarrhea)?

- How are my energy levels now, compared to what they were when I was "in good health"?
- Does my thinking feel "foggy" during the day?

You can probe as deeply as you'd like. My recommendation is to be honest with yourself whether your poor health is a direct result of poor life habits, choices, or actions. In essence, everything is. You're already feeling terrible. There's no point adding more to it. I give you permission to give yourself a break.

Modern medicine and practices are not a natural way of aging. They are not "inevitable entities" nor are they "just the way things are." It should not be common that everyone's grandparents are on 10 or more daily medications. Your life can be better. You deserve better. Let's get your health back!

"The doctor of the future will give no medicine but will interest his patients in the care of the human frame, in diet, and in the cause of prevention of disease."

— Thomas Edison

CHAPTER 5

THE NEW "OLD" SOLUTION: COMPOUNDING PHARMACY (PRECISION MEDICINE)

"We do not think ourselves into new ways of living, we live ourselves into new ways of thinking."

— Richard Rohr

The first question you might be asking yourself is, "What's a compounding pharmacy?"

It's a little like what makes up a great entree versus one that is just so-so. If you cook, you know what I mean. You can follow a recipe book to the letter and get a fairly decent dish out of the ingredients. You measure carefully using cups, teaspoons, and tablespoons, and you get a reliable result. But not one that a more confident chef will arrive at.

A good chef knows how to combine ingredients that you might not even consider. And in doing so, they can get more out of simple ingredients than you can. The same thing is true of a good compounding pharmacist.

The same standard of care of should go into compounding medications and nutrients for your individual biochemistry. And if you have a lot of questions about how that works, any doctor or healthcare provider should welcome those questions and answer them for you.

A medical specialist should also be able to take you, the individual, and come up with combinations of treatments unique to you, and ones that will result in the best outcomes as you make your journey to a healthier you.

The reality is that the more information gathered about a patient, the more precise the treatment for the patient becomes. With the methods outlined in Chapter 4, we at NutriChem are able to meet your needs.

However, what commonly takes place is that medical specialists recommend commercial products off the shelf, hoping these will match the patient. But when you function in a patient-centered care approach, you'll work with patients that have different, unique issues; therefore, your approach must be different for each one. You must match the product to the patient, not the other way around. And to do this means carefully compounding the right chemical solutions.

When we have a lot of information about the patient, the average drug does not treat patients with as much individualization as is possible. The average drug treats everyone as the same. Gather a group of one hundred people into a room. Some suffer from migraines, some from the flu, some bronchitis or strep throat, others broken bones, others sleep apnea or insomnia, others mood swings, hot and cold flashes, or mental disorders, and many will be treated with the same pill. This is the opposite of how we practice at NutriChem, which is *precision medicine*.

"Here, take this. This should make you feel better." This is an often-heard phrase in a normal medical office. Again, I want to reiterate that doctors do want to help you. They just haven't had the right tools or information at their disposal, but now they do. With the sheer amount of evidence pointing to the microbiome as the direct influence underlying all of these health problems, there is growing hope for patients with complex health issues.

Pharmaceutical companies have supported the traditional, older ways of thinking. Fortunately, a compounding pharmacy makes medications and supplements specific to the patient. As you become more knowledgeable about each individual patient, it's inevitable that the treatment also becomes more individualized for that patient. A compounding pharmacy is able to customize to *your* needs, not the other way around. Pharmaceutical companies customize medications and supplements according to *their* needs (which is all based on monetary profits and treating surface level symptoms).

Here are some examples of common compounds:

Problem	Compounding Solution
Dose of medication not commercially available	**Example: *Progesterone*** 100mg is the standard, commercially produced progesterone dosage. Some women only need 50mg of progesterone. We can make a custom 50mg dosage strength for those individuals.
Poor flavoring/child will not take medicine	We can add or change flavors to make medications palatable for children.
Sensitivity to fillers/ commercial ingredients	**Example: *Lactose*** Lactose is used as a filler in many commercially produced tablets. Many patients are lactose intolerant or sensitive to dairy, so they cannot have lactose. We can make pure medications or ones with substances that those with intolerances to commercial additives can take without adverse reactions.
Medication only produced as pills, and some patients cannot swallow pills	We can create a liquid form for patients that have trouble swallowing tablets or capsules
Limitations on how a medication can be administered	Some medications are only produced to be administered, for example, as rectal suppositories; we can formulate alternatives for different routes of administration.

A product is not made because it is not in high enough demand for a pharmaceutical company to produce it. These are called *"orphan drugs"*	We can compound small doses for individuals who have a need for specialized medications.
Reactions to existing creams on the market	Some creams and other topical applications are loaded with sensitizers which we can leave out.

NutriChem is also a National Association of Pharmacy Regulatory Authorities (NAPRA) compliant facility. In Ontario, it is mandatory to meet these high standards in order to compound. In the U.S., compounding pharmacies must adhere to United States Pharmacopeia (USP) standards.

Compounding pharmacies are a form of precision medicine.

At NutriChem, we're able to get more information about your genes and how they are affected by drugs, as well as how your genes affect the drugs. We're able to gather more information on your microbiome, nutrient status, and diet; therefore, our treatments must be individualized and precise. No one person or health issue is the same.

WHAT ARE SOME MORE BENEFITS OF COMPOUNDING PHARMACY?

This is another great question you should be asking your healthcare professionals. The overall benefit is better results with fewer side effects; better outcomes; and ultimately, less cost. This is because you're not just getting random pills or medications given to you to fix an issue, you're getting targeted results.

Remember, when you take Tylenol for a headache, your headache may go away, but without trying to figure out what the root cause may be (a poorly maintained microbiome, perhaps), your headache symptom will surface again and again. What you may really need is a specific kind of supplement or nutrient, but at a level highly specific to you. Maybe you don't need 1000 mg of vitamin C. Maybe you only need 100 mg. Maybe you're sensitive to certain chemicals and so you can't take anything that has those in them or you'll have a bad reaction and suffer more needlessly.

And then there are your genes. Genes react differently from person-to-person. Think of someone who is sensitive to gluten. Many medications don't take gluten intolerance into account. When we create a specific medication or supplement or nutrient-based program, we adjust it to fit an individual's specific needs.

And so, we might say, "Here is what you *really* need." And that's how our patients find lasting results. In addition, perhaps you're someone that needs a lower dose of the same kind of nutrient or supplement than someone else, but it needs to be combined in a specific way because you're sensitive to certain chemicals. Most general practice doctors will say, "Well, that isn't made or that doesn't exist." Naturally, you ask "Why not?" And the response, "It just isn't."

A pharmaceutical company's response might be, "That's too bad," but a good compounding pharmacy can and will help you by creating a specific nutrient or supplement or medication for your needs, even if they don't already exist.

THE PROCESS – HOW NUTRICHEM CREATES CUSTOM VITAMIN SUPPLEMENTS

The most cost-effective way to produce a vitamin is to measure the nutrient-based functions in your body. This tells us specifically what's happening within your unique biochemistry. We will take a look at your microbiome, look at the drugs that you're taking, look at your diet, your symptoms, your sex, your genetics, and your actual nutrient levels, and then give you a customized supplement specific to those requirements. And this is all based on research, evidence, and studies according to those specific parameters. No more guessing. It's time you found healing and started living your life fully.

This approach is super cost-effective. There are millions of people who take buckets of vitamins on a daily basis and see no results. I've had hundreds of patients come to my office and drop a huge box of multivitamin supplements on my desk. Despite all of these supplements and vitamins they take on a daily basis, they're still missing vital nutrients that are essential to them.

Many of these same people are the ones who are looking for the next trend or fad that they can latch onto and hope for results. This is why there are so many different diets out there, and so many different nutritional plans, and why no one sees lasting results. These same people never truly know what the root issue to their symptoms or health problems is: their microbiome. Our approach at NutriChem is anything but trendy. It is all-encompassing and scientifically enduring.

Your microbiome highly influences the nutrients that you absorb and the nutrients that your body uses. Your gut is working every day to maintain a balance. Every person's body requires something different. That's why it's crucial to do a full-body chemistry test to determine what is lacking or excessive in your body. For example, a female might need more or less of something than a male because their bodies are different.

It's all based on your genetics, your microbiome status, your diet, and how your body reacts and absorbs nutrients. It is vital that treatment is specialized according to the individual needs of each unique person.

Years ago, I would run lab tests on patients to determine what nutrient deficiencies they had. For example, I might have one patient who had an iron deficiency. So, we would develop a highly absorptive iron and just keep giving them more and more iron until their iron levels moved into the proper range. In time, as I researched and learned more about the microbiome, I realized that iron was only one factor. Anytime I measured nutrient levels and found them to be inappropriately low, it was often a direct result of an improperly functioning microbiome.

And whenever I corrected their microbiome, because the iron deficiency and the disrupted microbiome were married together, the results were dramatic, regardless of the dose of iron. This is how important the microbiome and the nutrient status is. These measurements not only tell you what you need to take, but they reveal where the trouble really is in relation to your absorption of nutrients.

However, it's interesting to know that some nutrients are sensitive to the microbiome. These include vitamin B12, iron, coenzyme Q10, magnesium, vitamin B6, and vitamin B1. I say that it's interesting because when you give someone a vitamin but it appears that it's not working or it's not increasing their nutrient levels, what do you do? Do you just keep giving them more and more vitamins or do you go deeper to find the root problem? When you do the latter, you almost always find that the issue is the microbiome.

WHAT ABOUT PATIENTS WHO CAN'T COME IN TO OUR OFFICE IN OTTAWA, CANADA?

Many of our patients are from all around the world. If they are not able to come in person, we usually correspond with them electronically or over the phone. This is common for many of the patients that I work with. A patient may call me from the United States and say, "Hey! I have a lot of gastrointestinal problems. How can I work with you?" And I might say, "I'd love to help you out," and ask, "Do you have any specific tests, such as lab work from your doctor, that show your B12, iron, or vitamin status?"

The first step is accumulating that data to determine a plan of action for them. Over the last thirty-five years, I've come to realize that even if

I don't have extensive lab results for the patient, and they have serious gastrointestinal problems, it's usually because there is a host of nutrient deficiencies as a direct result of an unhealthy microbiome.

In situations like these when someone can come to our main office in Ottawa, Canada, I'll say to them, "One of the most important things that I can do for you is to fix your gut." Naturally, this incites a slew of remarks from patients. They're calling about a mental disorder, or migraines, or insomnia, or depression or any number of other ailments, and here I am talking about their gut?

I go on to explain why I can't just give them customized vitamins. If they have an unhealthy gut, these vitamins will be less effective. We must correct the microbiome first before we can effectively correct nutrient deficiencies. That is why we create multivitamins that can bypass a disrupted microbiome while we fix it.

While we give them these multivitamins that can bypass their disrupted microbiome to adjust their deficiencies, we still need to fix their gut. We will always get better results with any vitamin when there is a healthier gut. The gut always comes first, even with nutrient status.

We also don't *need* testing in order to start repairing someone's gut. The full-body chemistry tests are useful to help pinpoint specific nutrient deficiencies within the body, but they're not always required. This is one reason why we are able to help people from all across the world. Sometimes when your gut is a mess, you don't need a specialized test to figure that out. So where do you start then? We can do a lot of work to repair someone's gut without much testing.

MICROBIOME DISRUPTION CHEAT SHEET

Your microbiome may be disrupted or compromised if you experience one or more of the following (this list is not exhaustive):

- Chronic low iron
- Chronic nutrient deficiencies (e.g. vitamin B12)
- Thyroid problems

- Adrenal problems
- Chronic constipation
- Diarrhea
- Irritable bowel
- Gas
- Bloating
- Nausea
- Vomiting after meals
- Burping
- Acid Reflux
- You're taking prescribed, over-the-counter, or illicit drugs
- PPIs (that fry your microbiome)
- Have you used a lot of antibiotics?
- You're eating a lot of processed foods
- You don't eat enough fruits and vegetables
- Prone to yeast infections
- Chronic fatigue
- Fibromyalgia
- Chronic skin conditions
- Inflammation problems in the brain, joints, or the gut
- Diabetes (Types 1 & 2)
- Chronic pain
- Brain Fog
- Anxiety
- Depression
- ADHD
- Addictions (food or drug)
- Resistant Weight Loss
- Obesity
- Severe Menopausal Symptoms
- Sleep Disorder
- Alzheimer's Dementia

Some of you might venture to say that we all have some of these problems. Well, yeah! There are so many culprits to these issues that people are unaware of. And our current understanding of medicine only exasperates the problem.

WHAT ABOUT PEOPLE BORN WITH THESE PROBLEMS?

The short answer is that the condition may be due to the microbiome that the infant inherits at birth. For a vaginal birth, the baby's microbiome is based on the mother's. For a C-section, it's based on the hospital's.

With a vaginal birth, you are transmitted the microbiome of your mother. If the mother has a healthy microbiome, the child will tend to inherit that healthy microbiome, and likewise, if the mother has an unhealthy microbiome, it is likely the infant will have an unhealthy microbiome. An unhealthy microbiome has been proven to affect brain and immune system development, and how your body interacts with the environment.

In the case of C-section infants, their microbiomes come from the hospital. Studies have shown that C-section babies are more likely to have allergies, skin conditions, and other health problems compared to vaginal birth babies because much of the immune system is developed in the digestive tract. A hospital is an allergic and biological disaster. In fact, in many countries, some providers give vaginal inoculations for C-section babies to provide healthy vaginal microflora from the mother. This is controversial, but the reason for this is because doctors are trying to manually transmit the mother's microbiome from the mother's vagina into the baby's mouth, skin, and digestive tract. However, we must be cautious with this because we don't want to transmit unwanted infections from mother to child either.

Doctors that perform vaginal swabbing are trying to mitigate the effect of the C-section birth on the infant. This is thought to lead to better health for C-section babies. The microbiome of the hospital is full of infections and is a very nasty environment. You have to think, the kinds of things that are able to survive in a hospital are very drug-resistant and pathogenic bacteria. A hospital can be a dangerous bacterial environment. So, imagine a C-section birth child when you run a microbiome test on them. Imagine what their results would be. Their microbiome is not just diminished, it's potentially extremely disturbed.

When doctors give the inoculation from the mother's vagina to the C-section baby, the microbiome of the mother could help to override the microbiome of the hospital. Hospitals in the UK and Europe are doing this, but every hospital all around the world should at least consider this practice for C-section births. The importance of the early microbiome on infants' health is so profound that we must try to set children up with a healthy microbiome from birth.

Whether this procedure is beneficial or not, it does display the growing awareness around the impact of the microbiome from birth.

WHAT WE USE IN OUR CUSTOM MULTIVITAMINS

As we dive deeper into the information about the microbiome, we're learning even more about the prevalence of deficiencies in the microbiome. For example, we find that roughly 75% of young women using normal oral contraceptives are vitamin B6 deficient, even when they're taking vitamin B6 in the form of pyridoxine. It actually has to be activated by the microbiome to produce activated B6, called P5P.

So even when women take vitamin B6, on average, we find that some of them are still deficient in vitamin B6. Many individuals who take supplements on a regular basis are still deficient because the microbiome is off. This is what can lead to symptoms like anxiety, depression, and inflammation.

We touched on it earlier. Vitamins or supplements will not help a person if the body cannot activate or absorb them via the microbiome. For this reason, NutriChem uses microbiome-safe and microbiome-independent nutrients. This means that the supplements or vitamins that we provide you can bypass the gut so that your body can absorb them even if your microbiome is disrupted. This helps alleviate your initial symptoms, but still requires for us to heal your gut.

For example, we use P5P as opposed to vitamin B6; we use benfotiamine as opposed to vitamin B1.

In this model, we give these patients the active form of these vitamins and supplements *as if they had an unhealthy microbiome and potential genetic issues* because this is the smart and safe way to approach their health. We avoid potential problems by using nutrients that do not rely on the microbiome or specific genetics to work. This approach has been proven to be effective. We use forms of nutrients that are better absorbed by the body and less dependent on a healthy microbiome.

Microbiome-Safe B vitamins:
- Pyridoxal-5-phospate (P-5-P) instead of vitamin B6
- Benfotiamine instead of vitamin B1. Benfotiamine is more fat-soluble and better absorbed than regular thiamine
- In severe cases, we use pure phosphatidylcholine instead of other choline forms, which bypasses choline metabolism in the microbiome. Phosphatidylcholine is a really important nutrient to bypass the microbiome

Microbiome-safe minerals:
- Potassium citrate (controlled-release)-helps alkalinize the small intestines, improving the pH levels
- Magnesium glycinate- a highly absorbable form of magnesium salt

Both affect the absorption of nutrients by the microbiome. No doctor or pharmacist should give medications, supplements, or nutrients without understanding their effects on the microbiome.

Prebiotic-soluble fibers:

Soluble fibers enhance a healthy microbiome and ultimately improve nutrient absorption.

There is so much evidence on the benefits of soluble fiber. So much evidence, in fact, that I would submit that there is nothing, of all of the products you could take or be prescribed by a pharmacy, including drugs and medication, with more evidence of having the ability to improve your longevity and quality of life than soluble fiber.

If there was only one health supplement that someone could ever take, it should be soluble fiber.

And this recommendation is different than saying, "You should take this vitamin or that vitamin." If soluble fiber could speak, it would say, "I've influenced all of your vitamins, I've influenced your brain, I've influenced your nutrient absorption, your blood sugar levels, your kidney function, your thyroid function, your liver function, your risks of developing any form of cancer." It all comes down to soluble fiber.

It's the nutrient that's most commonly lacking in the North American diet. And for some reason it appears to be hidden in grocery stores and pharmacies. Of all of the products that are provided and available, where do you find it? It should be front and center. Some examples of foods that are rich in water-soluble fibers include oats, beans, peas, seeds, and legumes.

WHAT A PATIENT VISIT MIGHT LOOK LIKE AT NUTRICHEM

The average person comes in and asks, "May I speak with someone?" They are curious, want help, and want to know what will make them feel better. However, skepticism arises when the answer isn't, "We have this easy solution," as people are conditioned to look for the next pill or other quick-fix. The other thing patients who come to NutriChem say when they walk in the door is, "Just tell me what to do." Most people are tired of the broken system that keeps them from feeling better. And they are willing to undergo anything.

We don't have a magic pill—there's no such thing—but what we do have is a time-tested, structured protocol to help us determine your underlying microbiome status.

That's why we encourage patients to do our Full-Body Chemistry test if they haven't already done lab work with their doctor. It's vital that we understand their gut and nutrient status. The test is the most cost-effective way to understand the full scope of a person's health.

The Full-body Chemistry test assesses the following:
- the gut bacterial strains present in the microbiome
- the metabolomics (the study of the set of metabolites within an organism, cell, or tissue) of their microbiome
- the organic oxidants
- the mitochondria
- all of their functional nutrient levels
- hormone levels
- sex hormone levels
- adrenal function
- thyroid Function
- vitamin & mineral status
- antioxidant status

- liver and kidney function
- iron
- Vitamin B12

After we perform this basic workup of their body, we sit down with them, with all of these tests in hand and review the results in conjunction with their symptoms.

Then we discuss with them what their primary issues are and what they want to achieve with treatment relative to what we see. From their perspective, most people come in already with a trained or conditioned medical viewpoint of their life. They might use phrases like, *my health problems, my headaches, my depression, my mood, I'm an alcoholic, I've got this problem, my son can't focus."* They present their symptoms like this.

This is only natural for patients to think this way since it's all they've ever been conditioned to think. For this reason, the first thing we do is review their microbiome status. We go over their gut bacteria and metabolomics. Metabolomics is the measurement of toxins or metabolites that come from the gut through analyzing their urine. After this, we're able to review their symptoms in relation to the likelihood of a damaged gut.

We use our **Body Health Pyramid** to assess the body.

Symptom
management

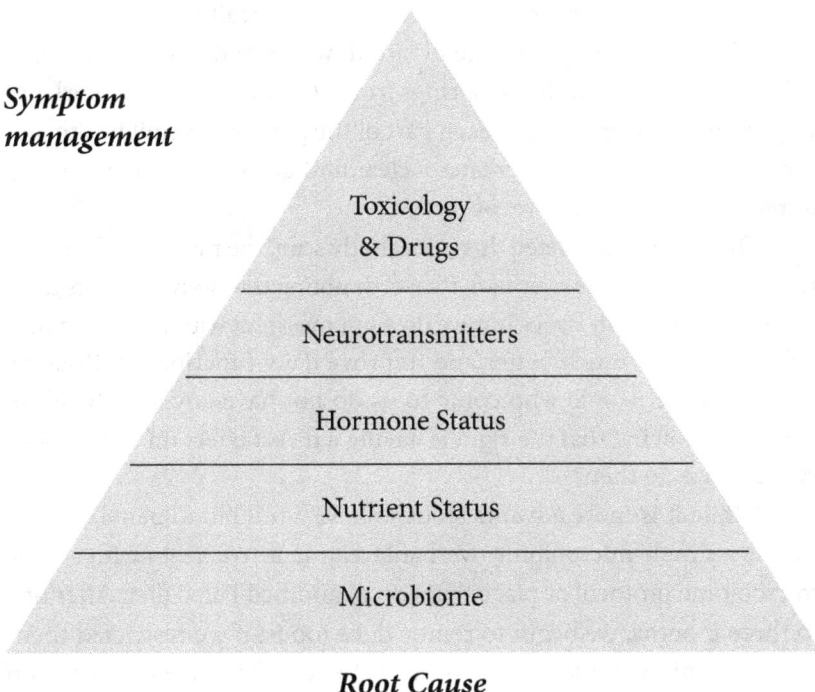

Toxicology
& Drugs

Neurotransmitters

Hormone Status

Nutrient Status

Microbiome

Root Cause

"Every brain has an optimal potential that should be unlocked."

The NutriChem philosophy relies on timelessness, the inevitability of science, and will never be trendy. The treatments we use at NutriChem are not going anywhere. *There is an inevitability of results.* Enduring treatments are possible when we work from enduring truths. This is the inevitability of the enduring basis of health. Hormones are not going anywhere. Nutrients like magnesium are not going anywhere. Hormones and nutrients will always be effective. And once you work with the basis of your biological system, your microbiome, you will have a certainty of results.

Your brain has an optimal potential that deserves to be unlocked. These are the proven foundations of brain health.

We start at the base of the pyramid, which is the microbiome, as this is where all life or illness springs from. Then we gradually work our way up to the tip, evaluating each part of the patient's overall health and their nutrient levels. This creates a clear and decisive roadmap of how to proceed to maximize recovery.

Once we've completed this initial body scan, the majority of patients require a microbiome overhaul. It's worth noting that some patients don't have obvious health issues but we do a gut overhaul with them and they still tend to feel much better and improve daily functioning. Roughly 60-80% of the people who come to us do not have any bloodwork or evidence showing that their gut is having a direct effect on their health. What do we do then?

While it is more advantageous to have a full blood panel, we can still do a simple microbiome overhaul treatment. We begin with a basic microbiome protocol or place them on a modified Paleo diet. After one to three months, we begin to reintroduce foods, if we restricted them. A healthy microbiome is then more resilient to food. We also insist on prebiotic fiber intake on a daily basis. This is nonnegotiable. We set up a maintenance diet that includes customized vitamins, fibers, probiotics, proteins, and/or fats (in case someone is not getting enough healthy fats in their diet).

THE RESULTS

In the first month, approximately 50% of our patients have significant improvements to their well-being and health. And I do not mean by a little bit. Their health symptoms and underlying conditions typically improve by 70% or more. It's people saying something like, "Oh my God! My life is SOOO much better! Thank you!"

It never gets old hearing the shouts of their breakthroughs or seeing the tears of joy. It's what we're here for.

For the other 50%, we dive deeper and have to spend more time killing off all the bugs and issues that are more resistant. Some patients are so sensitive or their microbiomes are so disrupted that in the first month, you have to start slow and be gentle as you kill off all the bad bacteria. They're so loaded with toxins that the kill-off effect would be too overwhelming for them. Think drug withdrawal. It's the same. So, we must take our time and be gentle for those severe cases.

If you can improve someone's health and life by 70% or more within the first month, why wouldn't more people do it? That's the million-dollar question! How do you convince someone that you have the solution to many of their health problems and get them to trust you and take action?

Ultimately, it will come down to whether you want to make a commitment to this path. Some people won't take action and will continue to struggle. This is understandable. Changing diet and lifestyle to improve the microbiome can be daunting. But the patients that do follow the plan that we lay out for them tend to see substantial improvements in their well-being and experience an abundance of life. The transformations can be astounding.

I had a patient once who had tried forty-one different antidepressants throughout her life. I'm not exaggerating. We had her do the Full-Body Chemistry test and were able to see where she was deficient, but her main concern was that I was going to rip her off of all of her medications abruptly. Even though she was miserable, she had become so dependent on those pills that they became her identity.

And when someone like me came around, who threatened to take that away, she resisted. Her thought was, "Why should I believe you? I've been taking forty-one antidepressants over the last thirty years of my life and none of them have helped. My gut is a mess. I feel like crap constantly. My digestive system is so disastrous, what makes you think that you can help?"

And I told her, as I tell many other patients who have the same concerns, "I am a pharmacologist. I'm actually a pharmacist. It's what I've been doing for over thirty-five years. I know what the drugs do better than anyone. If I knew of the forty-second antidepressant or pill that would change your life, I would give it to you. I'm not holding back."

The logical question would be, "How would the forty-second antidepressant help when the other forty-one haven't?" But I continue and say, "All I'm saying to you is that I'm going to fix your gut problem, which no one has addressed for the last twenty or thirty years. That's a long time! I'm going to fix your digestive problems, because it's been proven to affect your brain, and let's just see what's left."

And even though she had no choice and had no life as it currently stood, she still was holding on to the hope that the forty-second pill was going to be the one that came through and fixed all of her problems even though all of the evidence showed that those drugs weren't working and were actually causing a lot of her problems. For the life of me I just don't understand why anyone would want to live that way.

I actually asked her, "Ma'am, what am I missing here? What can I say that will convince you to take action and improve your health?"

And her response was the classic reaction, "How can you guarantee that I'm going to get better?"

BRAIN POWER TIP

Society has conditioned us to believe that we either win or lose. It's all or nothing, but this is not the case. Can I guarantee that she'll get better if we fix her gut? Yes, I can! I've helped thousands of patients before her do the same and the evidence proves it. All I can guarantee her, or any patient, is that I'll improve her digestive system and show the correlation between the gut and the mental disorders associated with it, which has been proven to be the case.

And I told her, "What's the risk in trying? Nothing else has worked. Why not try my way and see if it helps, even a little?"

Of course, I'm sympathetic with patients like her. I understand what they're going through. Life can be very bleak for patients like this. They're depressed, overwhelmed, run down, with all of their hopes betting on that next pill or quick-fix to solve all of their problems. She was overwhelmed by the concept that she was going to have to change her dietary habits. This can be scary for someone who's used to living a certain way; some can't even get to the grocery store because they feel so miserable all the time.

NutriChem is currently working on a partnership to deliver food to patients for those first thirty days. They no longer will have to worry about going to the store, what to buy, or what to eat and when. We provide it all for them. They simply just stick to the plan. What overwhelms people is the habit, not the science. They understand and even believe what I'm telling them, but they're afraid to let go. They'd rather hold onto the pain and suffering, even though it's killing them, than *feel* as though they have to give up a part of them.

I get it. It's hard when you're depressed, tired, hopeless, and feel like crap all of the time. The last thing you want to do is go to the store to stock up on foods you don't usually eat. It's difficult to change. But if you can beat the power of this false mindset, something great awaits you.

People think they have control over their lives, but not completely. I'm fighting the bad bacteria in their guts that's dictating their brain's behaviors and their lives. The irony in all of this is that we're addicted to crap that's affecting our guts, which then influences and dictates our behaviors, which then causes us to be resistant to change. It's that direct. When I try to come between someone and their cravings and addictions, even if they are unaware of it, it creates a huge resistance.

When you exhibit irrational behavior, like that woman did, who hoped that the next pill was going to solve her problems, it's usually because your gut chemistry is creating havoc on your brain and you're unaware of it.

Medications, or drugs, or food are causing these problems and very few people are aware of the connection.

While we understand that these cravings and addictions are a chemical issue, we label and blame people saying things like, "If you were just a stronger person, or if you went to AA, you would recover." But it's not something that can be tackled just at a personal level. The battle must be waged at the chemical level as well.

"Lots of people know what to do, but few people actually do what they know. Knowing is not enough! You must take action."

— Tony Robbins, #1 NYT bestseller of Unlimited Power

CHAPTER 6

HORMONES

"I have my hormones balanced.
Most doctors are giving women
synthetic hormones, which just
eliminate the symptoms, but it's
doing nothing to actually replace
the hormones you have lost.
Without our hormones, we die."

— Suzanne Somers

The #1 person that ever impacted NutriChem's use of hormones was Suzanne Somers. She actually came to Ottawa for an event with NutriChem on bioidentical hormones. She understood that women needed to know that they should not accept the "status quo". When she spoke in Ottawa, the response was overwhelming and the outcry from women to feel better during menopause was astounding.

When I met Suzanne Somers, it was gratifying to see that she embraced the notion that hormones have a direct impact on women's mental health. She understood the brain health of women and the importance of hormones with regard to brain function. She was speaking to other women and gathering information about how they felt. She understood that there were underlying problems. She could tell these issues went deeper and that just treating menopausal symptoms was not helping these women. Hormones actually help maintain the tissues of the body and brain. They are a fundamental treatment modality (see our pyramid) for health. Until Suzanne Somers became a spokesperson for this approach, women have just been managing symptoms. Many doctors still don't understand that using an antidepressant is not the same as using a hormone. The root cause for many women is lack of hormones, not lack of a medication. Suzanne Somers was a huge leader in the area of bioidentical hormones. Women trusted that she was onto something beyond just symptom management, and she often said that women should not accept the "status quo" in menopause. She asserted that menopausal women do not have to accept feeling poorly all the time.

Hormones are one of the most misunderstood and misused treatments in developed countries. It is crucial to know that all of these hormones are dramatically impacted by the microbiome. The four main groups of hormones found in both men and women are the thyroid hormones, the sex hormones, the adrenal hormones, and insulin.

Thyroid hormones come from the thyroid. The sex hormones come from the female's ovaries and the male's testes. The adrenal hormones come from your adrenal glands, and insulin comes from your pancreas. Every hormone secreted by one organ affects the rest of the body, whether in good or bad ways.

The most important concept of hormones that you should remember is that hormones are significantly affected by the microbiome.

Let's take your adrenal system as an example. Cortisol is your stress hormone, released by the adrenal glands. It triggers your stress response, like anxiety, affects body weight, insulin levels, as well as bone and heart health.

Every one of these hormones affects every other organ and system in your body.

HORMONE TREATMENT

Hormone treatments are very interesting because of the influence and relationship between them and the gut. The relationship between estrogens and the microbiome is known as the estrobolome.

This means that your gut bacteria affect the female hormone, estrogen. When you have an unhealthy microbiome, your body deconjugates and recycles estrogen, leading to higher estrogen levels. There are two direct adverse effects of an unhealthy gut and estrogen metabolism.

1.   Estrogen becomes more potent. Your healthy gut bacteria normally conjugate estrogen to allow it to be excreted through your urine. An unhealthy gut will have reduced conjugation, causing estrogen to recycle back into the body. In this way, you create higher and higher estrogen levels, which is associated with health problems.

2.   The body metabolizes estrogen into more potent forms that are more carcinogenic and harmful to the body. The consequence of this is significantly linked to hormonal imbalances, anxiety, insomnia, fertility issues, PMS, polycystic ovary system (PCOS) imbalances, and higher rates of breast cancer.

In men, an unhealthy microbiome increases estrogen metabolites and lowers active testosterone. Testosterone levels are suppressed by the high levels of estrogen circulating through the body that comes from body fat that is being re-circulated and re-conjugated back into the body. In other words, a disrupted microbiome in men can lead to excess estrogens, which ultimately suppress testosterone levels. This can lead to disastrous effects on men, causing fat gain, muscle loss, reduced energy and libido.

Dysbiosis in the gut can also over-activate the adrenal system. An unhealthy microbiome triggers higher levels of cortisol and also disrupts insulin levels to the point where the body can become insulin resistant. The microbiome can disrupt insulin sensitivity and other weight-regulating hormones, potentially causing Type 2 Diabetes and weight gain. Both high cortisol and dysregulated insulin adversely affect hormone status and directly compete with natural sex hormones like estrogen, progesterone, and testosterone.

You get a sort of triple whammy. A complex cascade of multiple hormonal problems arises when the microbiome is disrupted.

To make matters worse, this is compounded when you involve the thyroid and you don't metabolize thyroid hormones correctly either. Just to summarize, you can see how if the microbiome is disrupted, all of your hormonal systems can become disrupted. Before you take hormones, it's crucial to ensure your microbiome is healthy. All these things work together in a sort of network. Each hormone influences the other and the microbiome basically regulates all of it.

MENOPAUSE, PMS, & HORMONAL IMBALANCES

I had a patient once who said she rung out her bed sheets every night from sweat and lost seven pounds of water from the severity of her hot flashes. This had been going on for years before she even began menopause. This was a clue that she had a serious issue with her microbiome.

The first plan-of-attack was fixing that.

By reviving her microbiome, we calmed her adrenal system, which reduced the hot flashes. Before she came to me, she used different hormones to treat her symptoms. These helped a little, but they never addressed or influenced the root cause of her hot flashes: the microbiome.

Cortisol was the dominant hormone impacting her microbiome. Cortisol is the main stress hormone, secreted by the adrenal glands, and if it is excessively high for long periods, it dampens the levels and effects of almost all of the other hormones. She could not get a result from her sex hormones until her cortisol was reduced, and this required fixing her microbiome. When we healed her microbiome, her digestive problems improved, which reduced the cortisol levels, which then dramatically stopped her hot flashes.

Once we were able to do that, we could address adding estrogen and progesterone (in low doses) to get the lasting results we wanted.

For her, the disrupted microbiome caused all of her problems, but she kept taking hormones, thinking this was solving the problem. They never worked very well because no one understood the relationship between the microbiome and the symptoms of menopause (hot flashes and sweat).

The microbiome is highly involved with these symptoms. If we take a woman with PMS or menopause, and she has a healthy microbiome, her transition will be smoother because her adrenal system is not overly engaged, it's not overactive, or hypersensitive due to a disrupted microbiome.

But a woman with an unhealthy microbiome with the added stress of daily life will cause her adrenal system to become highly sensitized. Her hormone levels will become more erratic and will send her into a tailspin of serious menopausal symptoms.

If we were to only give her hormones, they would work, but my experience is that you will have a wide variation of how much you need to give someone to warrant a specific result. Where one woman may only need ten milligrams of progesterone, another may need three hundred. But why?

In my experience, the woman with the healthier microbiome requires less while the more disrupted microbiome requires more. Menopausal women tend to enjoy gentler and more sustainable results with lower doses of hormones when their microbiome is healthier. When we approach the gut first, we typically obtain more consistent results with lower doses of hormones. There's a clear relationship between the microbiome and estrogen hormone levels, and it's known as the estrobolome.

THE TYPICAL HORMONAL IMBALANCES FOR PATIENTS

Over the last thirty-five years, a term I often hear is estrogen dominance.

All this means is that women have too much estrogen and too little progesterone. That's the number one issue I see in female hormone patients who come to me. So, while it may appear that some women have too much estrogen and not enough progesterone, especially during menopause, this is not the main problem. The microbiome is highly involved in neutralizing estrogen. If you don't have a healthy microbiome, you'll be more likely to experience estrogen dominance. This leads to a wider range of menopausal symptoms and accounts for why some women experience menopausal symptoms even before they go through menopause. Differing estrogen levels created by the microbiome leads to a wide variety of menopausal symptoms in women.

This is also why women in some non-industrialized countries tend to have fewer menopausal symptoms. They have healthier microbiomes, healthier diets, and other factors in their lives resulting in fewer hormonal imbalances and symptoms. These women exhibit fewer fertility issues, less PMS, and more tolerable menopausal symptoms.

Because they have a healthier microbiome, their hormones are far more balanced, their adrenal system is engaged properly with the management of hormones, their thyroid functions better, and the rest of their body functions better as well. For more than 30 years, I've been asking the same question about estrogen dominance: "Why is it happening and what's causing it?"

We now finally have the answer: it's the unhealthy substances that we put into our bodies which interfere with our microbiome's ability to metabolize hormones.

SYNTHETIC VERSUS BIOIDENTICAL HORMONES

It's pretty straightforward. The female body makes estrogen and progesterone. We've known about the forms of estrogen and progesterone that the human female body produces for over seventy years. And then, all of a sudden, we began giving women synthetic hormones for commercial reasons.

Pharmaceutical companies began patenting synthetic and semi-synthetic hormones that aren't naturally found in a woman's body. These synthetic hormones attempt to mimic human progesterone and estrogen.

The results have been unsuccessful and harmful. In the *Women's Health Initiative Study*, the biggest one ever done, it was shown that in the group that used synthetic estrogen and progesterone, it was the synthetic progesterone that caused an increased risk of breast cancer. Every study that has examined synthetic progesterone has always linked it to an increased risk of breast cancer. Studies have shown that women with lower levels of natural progesterone have higher rates of breast cancer. Not only does synthetic progesterone increase the chances of breast cancer, it causes disruptions to sleep, increased cholesterol, is hard on the heart, and has more adverse effects. Compare this to bioidentical, human female progesterone, which reduces cholesterol, builds bones, stabilizes the heart and the central nervous system, and is responsible for a more balanced sleeping pattern (it's what allows for women to sleep).

So why on earth would anyone use synthetic progesterone? It's not logical, and yet, it's still being prescribed to people, and we wonder why we have so many problems.

Synthetic progesterones, such as medroxyprogesterone, are dangerous, carcinogenic, and should not really be considered "hormones" at all in the medical market. Medroxyprogesterone is not the same as progesterone! All progesterones are not the same. I've been saying this for thirty years, but now mainstream medicine is finally acknowledging that fact, and is shifting toward the trend of prescribing bioidentical progesterones and estrogens.

However, even to this day, I still come across women that are being prescribed synthetic hormones. I had a woman just yesterday come in to see me who was prescribed synthetic progesterone. She had sleep problems, and of course the first thing that I recommended for her was to get off this poisonous nonsense and onto something that would actually solve her sleep problems and reduce her risk of breast cancer.

As for the difference between synthetic and bioidentical hormones, it would be like asking, "What is the difference between horse hormones and human hormones?" It's a crazy question, but you have to still ask it because we still have pharmaceutical companies creating and prescribing these harmful hormones. And I would say, "We have less problems with human hormones, as you might expect."

This seems like common sense, that we would respond better to hormones from our own species. Similarly, as our knowledge has advanced, we've migrated to human insulin from pork insulin, because there are less side effects associated with human insulin. It makes sense that women respond better to human hormones than hormones from another organism.

When it comes to pre-menopausal or menopausal women, they should only use bioidentical (human) hormones. Generally, bioidentical hormones work best if applied transdermally through the skin because they require lower dosages compared to oral dosing, they better mimic natural blood levels, and they pose less risk of blood clots in the case of estrogens.

Interesting fact:
You can reduce the amount of estrogen that you use by ten times when you apply it through the skin.

BRAIN POWER TIP

If you improve the microbiome's health, you can improve every single woman's hormonal imbalances. I will add though that some women may still require additional support and that's when you use a little bit of direct bioidentical hormone to fix something like vaginal dryness, hot flashes, sleep disturbances, or bone loss. Improving the microbiome can improve hormonal symptoms in women, and if you do use bioidentical hormones, it is easier for them to eliminate symptoms if they have a healthy microbiome.

You fix the microbiome first, then you address the hormones. You don't just slap a hormone patch on a woman and say, "There you go! You're cured!" It doesn't work that way necessarily. You won't get the same results that you would if you improved a woman's microbiome and THEN administered hormones as needed.

It all goes back to the Body Health Pyramid. The microbiome is the foundation that everything else is built upon. If you have a faulty base, your edifice can topple. When a storm blows, the pieces on the top begin to fall or crack first.

Hormones are the safer method to deal with hormonal imbalances, but only when you use bioidentical hormones, and even more effectively, when you use them in conjunction with a microbiome overhaul.

Even if you never knew about the microbiome and the importance it plays on your overall health, bioidentical hormones are safer and more effective than synthetic hormones. It's a no brainer. They just plain work.

"To keep the body in good health is a duty...otherwise, we shall not be able to keep our mind strong and clear."

— Buddha

CHAPTER 7

DIET

"Your diet is a bank account. Good food choices are good investments."

— Bethenny Frankel

Diet is the single most important factor for good health. People are unaware of the implications of what they consume and how it's affecting their body and mind.

A question that I get often from patients or people curious about NutriChem and our protocols is, "What diet regimen do you give patients?"

And I explain to them about the diet of the brain. In the last thirty-five years, we've evolved to understand that what you eat affects your brain. This originated with patients who suffered from seizure disorders being given the ketogenic diet. In many cases, the ketogenic diet, which contains little to no carbohydrates, actually stopped their seizures. Similarly, we have also used dairy-free, gluten-free, low FODMAP, and specific carbohydrate diets in a variety of medical conditions with some success.

We don't know exactly why these diets work for these conditions, but we do know that they are strongly associated with significant shifts in the microbiome. The food shift leads to a microbiome shift that can, for example, change the seizure activity in children's' brains.

And what's interesting is that when all of these diets first originated, they were considered alternative solutions, and doctors would "pooh-pooh" them. However, parents were doing these on their own. And then finally, of course, these diets and ways of thinking were adopted and have since been utilized in traditional medical practices for treating brain issues.

This is exciting. We're in a new evolutionary stage in terms of understanding that what you eat affects the way your brain works. Does the ketogenic diet work because you're making ketones and shifting the acid-base balance of the body, or is it due to a microbiome shift? We now know through studies that the effect is not due to the acid-base shift or ketones alone, so what is the cause? It appears to be the microbiome shift.

What's key is to realize that when you use or shift any food intake, you're in fact dramatically altering your microbiome. Any food shift changes your microbiome. When we get into a plethora of different diets out there, it's crucial to understand that any diet shift will change your microbiome. And once again, this microbiome shift can have a significant impact on the brain.

The most powerful and effective shift is to remove processed foods, such as those full of sugar or preservatives, or foods containing chemicals like pesticides, antibiotics, growth hormones, and artificial flavoring. Basically, eradicate all of the junk that is not whole food. Once you remove these from your diet, replace them with non-chemically enhanced fruits, vegetables, and meat. That is, make sure there has been no use of pesticides, hormones, or antibiotics in their growing or raising.

This sounds obvious, but in my years of experience, making this change exacts one of the most immediate shifts and triggers a response resulting in improvement of the body and mental health in about 50% of the cases. So, a shift in diet is just recalibrating what people intake.

Within an inflamed gut, the majority of people have a disrupted microbiome. In those individuals, things like sugar, dairy, gluten, or certain grains are also more prone to cause trouble in an already inflamed microbiome. This triggers things like a leaky gut, which causes inflammatory substances to leak into your body.

There are a few different levels of diets that we implement with our patients.

For the first level, we usually recommend a modified paleo diet, which is essentially removing all processed foods, added sugars, dairy, and gluten, and then supplementing that with only whole foods, fruits, and vegetables. Generally, we remove grains and anything that would not be found in an ancestral, hunter-gatherer diet, such as sugar, dairy, gluten, and alcohol.

That's the first level and should be the first level for almost anyone. The evidence shows that a 30-day shift—and often sooner—is enough to make a dramatic and significant change in your microbiome. And we have found this can have a profound impact on the body and the brain in multiple direct and indirect ways.

So, shifting to a basic Paleolithic-style diet is the first step. If people require more after about 30 days, then we go deeper because sometimes people have done minor modifications and their microbiome is so inflamed that we actually have to go down another layer.

We do these shifts in 30-day increments. We do this because the evidence shows that thirty days is enough to make a significant change in your microbiome with food.

Depending on your practitioner and your symptoms, we may then go to an anti-inflammatory or low FODMAP diet. This is the next level down. We remove certain additional fruits and vegetables from your diet that have been shown to grow or disrupt your microbiome in certain ways.

Most people are unaware of the low FODMAP diet. A low FODMAP diet refers to low fructose, oligosaccharides, disaccharides, monosaccharides, and polyols. You don't need to know what these are other than that they are sugars found in certain fruits and vegetables that some people have trouble digesting and so they can disrupt their microbiome. These sugars can cause a lot of gastrointestinal distress and people tend to get relief when they are removed from their diet.

The key point to take away from a low FODMAP diet is that we are essentially removing specific sugars from certain fruits and vegetables. Again, this has been proven to be one of the most effective things in the treatments for irritable bowel syndrome (IBS). Naturally, the most effective and official therapy used for IBS is the low FODMAP diet, and the low FODMAP diet is a microbiome-altering diet.

By removing certain sugars that feed or fuel specific inflammatory gut bacteria, you're in essence starving out the bad bacteria. I want to emphasize that it usually only takes thirty days to see positive results with dietary changes. And when I say positive results, I'm talking a significant and dramatic improvement in gastrointestinal and mental health issues. There is a clear trend toward consistent and inevitable improvement with microbiome shifting diets. After the initial 30-day diet, if people have improved, we can slowly start to re-integrate foods, one at a time, back into their diet.

When I'm speaking to patients, I usually describe this process and situation as two mountains. On the one mountain, you have bad bacteria and a disrupted microbiome and all of the health problems that come with it. The other mountain is a healthy microbiome with no health or mental problems and the freedom to eat and do whatever you like (within moderation).

The process is taking people down from the bad mountain and over to the good. When we alter or adjust their diet, we're essentially taking them off of the bad mountain and into the valley. Once there, we continue to kill off the unhealthy bacteria while simultaneously feeding and restoring the good bacteria with probiotics and soluble fibers.

For those patients or people who do not continue to restore their microbiome, they remain in the valley. This is where you are beginning to do better, but now you have to follow all of these strict food restrictions. You can eat this but can't eat that. And you're stuck in this miserable state.

The goal is to get people from the bad mountain to the good mountain. That's where a healthy microbiome and an abundant life reside. This is where there is very little food restriction, and your microbiome is resilient enough to withstand the challenges of a modern, varied diet. Evidence is mounting that the increasing food sensitivities we are seeing is just a symptom of disrupted microbiomes.

Some patients ask if we provide different diets for different symptoms or health issues or diseases. The answer is no. The world says that there's a diet for everything. If you suffer from seizure disorders, inflammation, or obesity, just get on this diet or take this pill. But that's not how it works. Ultimately, there is no perfect diet, but any diet we use will remove processed foods, like refined sugar, dairy, gluten, alcohol, artificial sweeteners, preservatives, and antibiotics.

What's amazing is that the human microbiome can be healthy with huge extremes of natural foods. For example, some people have an all protein diet and can be very healthy, and others consume a vegetarian or vegan diet and can be very healthy. And it is the microbiome that is the master regulator in this variation. It can adapt to allow you to digest and metabolize a huge array of foods. But what the microbiome cannot handle is crappy modern junk food!

The human gut can handle almost any natural molecule, but it cannot tolerate synthetic chemicals it never evolved to handle. The microbiome is a great adaptor for whatever diet nature can throw at you, but it cannot adapt to our current processed foods or a hostile modern environment. The rainforest of the microbiome can become a dying wasteland of bad bacteria with overexposure to a modern, industrialized, junk food diet.

What is the perfect diet? It varies from individual to individual, but certain general rules apply: you always have to remove processed foods like refined sugar, alcohol, dairy, gluten, artificial sweeteners, preservatives, and antibiotics. In the acute healing phase of any diet, you may have to restrict certain foods to rapidly eradicate certain overgrown bad bacteria. We call this the "weeding" phase of our diets.

Using a specific diet for a specific condition is the old-school way of helping people. It's the same approach that doctors take with drugs. If you have this specific symptom or condition, you will get this specific drug. If you have this specific illness, maybe you can use this specific diet to help with it. We try to make it overly simple by saying something like, "Okay, what's my food or what's my drug or what's my special regimen that I need to take away, add, or adjust to feel better?" Meanwhile, somewhat general dietary shifts such as removing processed junk, can have a dramatic impact in ~50% of people on the microbiome within 30 days. For the other 50%, further dietary changes or specific probiotics and prebiotics will be required.

Human allergy testing is similar. If someone takes an allergy test and finds out that they are allergic to forty things, does this mean that they are actually allergic to forty foods, or is it just a symptom of a disrupted microbiome and an inflamed gut, which is now reacting to all of these foods?

Another question that I generally get asked is, "Do patients only eat what I tell them to or can they just add supplements and a dietary plan to what they're already eating?"

Anyone that has a microbiome problem would ideally shift their food intake. I've had some people ask, "Can I just take some fiber or probiotics?" Probiotics and fiber can help, but the best results come from a dietary shift. If you change your diet, you generally change all of the major bacterial structures in the microbiome, whereas when you use a probiotic or fibers, you only change a small fraction of the bacterial structures in your microbiome.

Diet is the most effective method, but probiotics and prebiotics can help "nudge" the microbiome in the right direction. Probiotics and especially fibers (prebiotics), can really "lock" in the changes to the microbiome we make via diet.

I must note that I have some patients that cannot or will not change their diets, and they can get results with probiotics and fibers, but ideally, they would get the most out of a diet change. I acknowledge that with some of my patients, especially children, this is impossible though. We do what we can with probiotics and fibers in these cases, and they help, but I know that they could get more benefit from dietary changes.

The root goal is that you want to change the entire forest, not just individual trees. You need to change and alter the entire environment. It's difficult to do this without changing what you intake via diet. And when people finally get a grasp on this concept, they exclaim, "Oh! So, it's the food I'm eating?" And I say, "Yes! You are finally getting it."

I don't say this last bit quite as frankly, but I get the point across. Food is vital to your health, not just survival. So, we may restrict your diet depending on what your symptoms are and your ability to handle certain things. Some people with the most severe complications and the worst eating habits have more severe withdrawals when we implement a new diet. Treating these patients can actually be like dealing with addiction patients. The bad bacteria in their gut have actually hijacked their brain's reward systems, producing cravings for junk foods that promote their own survival. These people can have severe withdrawal reactions from processed foods. Despite their severe reactions, we don't need to do anything dramatic in their diets to elicit a big change in their health.

We don't have to do a lot of work. Some people have already done a lot of work before they come see us. I had someone just the other day who had done a restrictive dairy and gluten-free diet. She ate clean but still had severe stomach and mental health problems. We adjusted her diet to a low FODMAP diet because she had already done the first level of food restriction and wasn't getting any results. When we made this small shift, she had dramatic results.

After this happened, we locked in those changes with fiber and probiotics, and then slowly began to reintegrate different food groups into her diet. We did this one at a time. This process is what I like to call shifting a patient from the bad mountain to the good mountain.

WHAT ABOUT EXERCISE DURING THIS PROCESS?

This is another interesting topic for discussion because when I first started working with patients, I mentioned the need for exercise all the time. But today, as we fix their microbiome, their energy levels shoot up, their mood elevates, and they begin to tell me that they are now exercising. They tell me they are more active now than they've been in their entire lives. There are still those rare situations where a patient's activity does not increase. I would say one out of every ten people who come to see me for help does not see an increase in their activity output. This is not due to lack of improved health; instead, it's a direct correlation from their habits that cause this sedentary lifestyle.

The funny thing is that when people start feeling better they begin exercising more. In most cases, it takes very little encouragement from me. Obviously, exercise has been proven to give you a healthier microbiome. And so, the more that you move or the more active that you are, the healthier your body will be. Exercise improves your gut chemistry. How cool is that?!

WHAT DO PEOPLE DO AFTER THE FIRST 30 OR 60 DAYS?

I want to reiterate that we go with increments of thirty days to get these dramatic shifts in health improvement. Our ultimate objective is 100% resolution of gastrointestinal problems no matter how long this takes.

However, 50% of our patients do so within the first thirty days. Others may take sixty or ninety days. The time does not matter so long as we fix the problem. Our objective is not minor resolution of gut problems, but major improvement or resolution of all gut problems.

This is our gut protocol. We go down diet-by-diet and product-by-product until we achieve 100% resolution of the gastrointestinal problems. When we do, we now know that we have a healthy and sustainable microbiome.

We've also found that this has a direct correlation to a significant improvement in mental health issues. Once we reach 100% resolution, we enter into the "gut maintenance" phase. That is, we lock in this improvement with the appropriate probiotics and soluble fibers. Next, we slowly bring back a more varied diet. The evidence actually shows that a healthy microbiome is more resistant and resilient to "crappy" foods. However, I've noticed that those who have experienced a full resolution of their gut and mental health disorders have now developed a deeper understanding of their tolerance for certain foods and begin to live with healthier lifestyles in general. Linking back to addiction, these people have broken their chemical addiction to crappy foods. Now they are ruling their microbiome, their microbiome is not ruling them.

And now we don't even need tell them to restrict their diets. Ironically, our objective is not to restrict your diet, but to increase the variety of healthy foods you can eat, and to improve your awareness of the impact of that food on your body and brain.

WHAT SHOULD YOU DO NOW TO MAINTAIN YOUR HEALTHY MICROBIOME?

With your increased awareness of processed foods and their impact on your body, you're more acutely aware of how important fruits and vegetables are to your gut ecosystem–even more so the importance of food without chemicals, pesticides, or antibiotics. Potentially, you may be more aware of sugar, dairy, and gluten in highly processed foods and how they affect your body. But the important thing for you to take away is that your diet is no longer restricted. It was never truly restricted, just off balance. You can have fun with some junk food, but just don't go back to the way you were. In your illness, you felt depressed over gaining weight because you were unaware of the impact that the food and products that you were eating were having on your body. You learn through your healing not to go there again.

The other day, I had a former patient freaking out because he ate a couple slices of pizza. Naturally, I laughed, but this is a real fear that many people have. I just told him that it was okay and that he could have fun now that his microbiome was healed. A resilient microbiome can handle it (in moderation)! A healthier gut gives you more options, not less options.

The problem moving forward with developing healthy habits is not so much about the habits as it is with the food. We've been conditioned to believe that food is not the problem and is not important by these trillion-dollar food industries. Everyone says that they have a healthy diet, but no one really knows what a healthy diet really means.

I had a kid come to me once with severe mental health problems and the parents and the kid said things like, "I saw my psychiatrist and he told me that it was pointless to come to see you because you can get everything you need from your diet."

This gave me pause because the kid was drinking nothing but Red Bull energy drinks all day long, which have been proven to inflame your brain. My response to him was, "Did your psychiatrist ask what you were ingesting each day?" He said no. I then went on to explain to him how what we intake affects our brain and our body.

While this is an extreme example, when I ask people if they consume healthy food, almost 99% say, "Yes, of course!" However, upon actually investigating their diet, it becomes very apparent that 99% of them are not eating anything approaching healthy food. Their diets are often very low in fruits, vegetables, and soluble fibers, and very high in junk food, caffeine, sugar, and alcohol. It is common in traditional medicine to hear the phrase, "You can get all of your nutrients in your diet," yet I have never heard of a conventional healthcare provider actually asking a patient, "What are you eating in your diet?" I hear the first statement so often, but no one follows that up with, "And what does your diet consist of?" A patient should always try to have a serious discussion about diet with their doctor.

Sometimes what you see is so extreme and distorted from the reality of the situation.

I had another woman who ate a lot of junk food. Her diet did not include fruits or vegetables, and as it turned out, she was highly sensitive to even minor dietary adjustments. I didn't give her any products. I merely said, "Let's start gently by removing the junk from your diet. Let's take away the processed foods, chemicals, and diet drinks, and begin to give you fruits and vegetables. Let's just clean this up."

She had terrible reactions to these changes including anxiety, pain, and stomach upset. She called me and said, "You're hurting me!" And I said, "I can't hurt you by taking crap out of your diet and feeding you fruits and vegetables. Your microbiome is so distorted that literally your behavior and addiction are a direct result of these bad bacteria trying to signal for you to eat more junk food. The dying bad bacteria are triggering your cravings for junk foods in order to fuel their own survival, because you've stopped feeding them."

As I've said before, inflammatory bad bacteria need the junk to survive. If your body is used to consuming a lot of crap, when you remove this, you will experience some mild withdrawal symptoms similar to those of a drug addict. This is just those bad bacteria trying to convince you to eat more of the stuff that feeds them so that they don't die.

It is a new concept to a lot of people, the idea that such symptoms are similar to addiction withdrawals. Some people find it hard to wrap their head around, like this woman, but when the epiphany strikes, you will gladly starve the bad bacteria and reclaim what is rightly yours.

BRAIN POWER TIP

Anything in life worth doing is worth doing right. As you learn about your microbiome and work to restore it, you will face obstacles and become tempted to quit. Perhaps you'll feel as though your health problems are getting worse. While this is not the case, it still does not dissuade the real emotion and physiological response that you're experiencing.

But don't lose heart. Thousands of people have made this journey and have gone through the exact same thing and are now living healthy, free lives. Think about your health like you do about your career or finances. If someone walked up to you today and said, "In less than thirty days, if you follow these instructions, you will have one million dollars," would you listen to them? Would you follow the instructions even if they didn't always make sense? What is your health worth to you? One million dollars? Two million dollars? Or, would you quit when it got tough, seemed like it wasn't working, or because others were telling you to quit? People will do a lot for money, but what will they do for their health?

Some give up and miss out on the experience and the endless possibilities of a happy, healthy life. Others will never try, and will remain where they are or become worse, envying those on the other mountaintop.

Thirty days seems like a long time when you really want something, but it's tiny in the large scheme of things. Your health is the same. Commit to rebooting your health in thirty days and see how much better your life is. You won't regret it.

"If you don't like something, change it. If you can't change it, change your attitude."

— Maya Angelou

CHAPTER 8

PROBIOTICS

"The health benefits for which probiotics can be applied include conditions such as gastrointestinal infections, certain bowel disorders, allergy, and urogenital infections, which afflict a large portion of the world's population. The application of probiotics to prevent and treat these disorders should be more widely considered by the medical community."

— Joint FAO/WHO Expert Consultation,
Codex Alimentarius Commission

Before we dive into probiotics, let's recap on the structure of the microbiome.

The microbiome consists of trillions of cells and is a complex mini ecosystem that determines your overall mental and physical health. 10,000-15,000 different species of bacteria exist within the human gut. Approximately 75% of these bacteria are considered anaerobes, which means that if they are exposed to oxygen, they will die. Thus, we cannot give a bunch of these probiotics in capsule form as a supplement. For this reason, administering probiotics is only marginally effective.

We grow most of the good bacteria with fiber. We can only impact the microbiome so much with probiotics because the majority of the beneficial bacteria are destroyed by oxygen. To increase these specific beneficial bacteria, we have to feed them with specific fibers. Despite this limitation, probiotics still have their place, based on evidence that proves their effectiveness in gut recovery.

Many clinical studies have proven that the microbiome is incrementally impacted even by small doses of probiotics. I say small to insinuate the fact that if there are trillions of bacterial cells living within the microbiome, then what would a million or a billion be in comparison? And yet, even something small improves the microbiome significantly. Sometimes just nudging the microbiome in the right direction is effective. It just wants to be healthy!

HOW DO PROBIOTICS IMPACT THE MICROBIOME?

Scientific research approaches the microbiome through a reductionist method. This method is a very powerful tool, but it does not necessarily capture the larger complexity and power of the microbiome. This means that we examine each strain of bacteria within specific conditions. An example of this is that certain harmful bacteria are more prevalent in the microbiomes of people with certain diseases. Like pharmaceutical companies, we use these strains of bacteria to pinpoint specific biochemical effects. But we must be careful not to only look at the trees, and miss the forest. We must look at the whole ecosystem that is the microbiome.

We are always looking for specific bacteria to account for specific diseases, such as behavioral issues in down syndrome, or autism, or depression, for example. My own research has revealed that in autism certain strains of more harmful bacteria tend to be more prevalent. Even animal research has shown that we can transfer diseases between hosts (animal-to-human or human-to-human) through the microbiome. Pharmaceutical companies have created patented forms of bacteria that target improvement of mood, or diarrhea, or lower cholesterol, for example.

So, we're always looking to find that one bacteria to solve a specific problem. This reductionist thinking has conditioned us to think that there's a special bacteria or "magic" microorganism that will fix all of their problems. This research on specific species is very exciting and helpful. However, it is an understanding of the diversity and interrelationships of all of the organisms that has the most potent effects. Reductionist thinking is a common misconception that we've been led to believe, but it is an oversimplification of the potential of the microbiome as a whole. It would be like trying to improve a rainforest with only one type of tree, when what we need is a whole group of plants, trees, grasses, and shrubs to truly transform the microbiome. And of course, the microbiome is much more complex than that. As a pharmacist, I love running a specific study on a specific bacteria in a specific condition, but this does not capture the complex ecosystem that is the microbiome.

As a chemist, I would love to find that one substance that will solve all your health problems. But this is a flawed perception of reality.

For instance, certain bacteria metabolize phosphatidylcholine differently, which then alters what this nutrient does in the body. This could turn an essential nutrient into a very harmful substance. Phosphatidylcholine is an important and beneficial nutrient in the body. Among its many attributes, it plays key roles in cognition and liver function. However, if phosphatidylcholine is metabolized by bad bacteria in the gut, then trimethylamine oxide (TMAO) is produced. High levels of trimethylamine oxide are associated with cardiovascular events like heart attack and stroke. This is a double negative, because if you have an unhealthy microbiome, you are not only absorbing less phosphatidylcholine, you are metabolizing it into harmful substances. So, a commonly beneficial nutrient like phosphatidylcholine can be rendered harmful by an unhealthy microbiome. A Mediterranean diet, for example, can help make phosphatidylcholine good for you, whereas a poor diet will make it worse for you and increase your risk of heart disease and other health problems. Phosphatidylcholine paired with a very healthy microbiome-friendly diet (such as the Mediterranean diet) is great for you, but choline paired with an unhealthy diet full of junk food is potentially harmful.

So even if one molecule is usually beneficial, its interaction with the microbiome can alter it so that it has a negative effect on you. This makes having a healthy microbiome even more important for sustained health because the type of strains of bacteria in the gut hugely influence our metabolism of virtually all nutrients.

As a pharmacist, I'm always reviewing reactions to chemicals and calculating subtle changes that occur when different interactions take place. So, when someone comes in with health problems, I can create customized probiotics or bacteria specific to their health problems. This is because there is a ton of evidence that links specific bacteria to either improved or worsened health. But this reductionist method is limited. You can only do so much with a probiotic when there is a disrupted microbiome.

No matter how much you try to influence one piece of the entire structure, if you don't know the entire environment or structure of your gut, you're missing all of the potential benefits of having a healthy microbiome. This is why you cannot take one pill to solve all your problems. You may find it helped a little bit, but it didn't solve the entire root issue. For example, I have had patients with alcohol use disorder, and I have used psychobiotics (probiotics that affect mental health) that dramatically reduced their cravings for alcohol. So, you see, one probiotic can bring change to your chemistry, but it won't likely solve everything.

"Probiotics provide an extra layer of strength. (They behave like) soldiers in your intestinal tract to combat pathogens . . ."

— Dr. Mary Ellen Sanders

But I must reiterate that diet is the real backbone of a microbiome shift. Probiotics accelerate recovery, but their effects are limited without changing the diet and taking soluble fiber. Most of the probiotic products that you find on the shelves of stores and pharmacies are different combinations of lactobacillus and/or bifidobacterium. Whenever we formulate specific bacteria for a specific problem, we deliver these in much higher doses to stimulate more rapid recovery. Many of the probiotic products we use aren't found at your typical health food store or pharmacy.

People want results fast. This poses a real issue for us when patients come in with a problem. They are expecting quick recovery and we have to try to figure out a way to make that possible. It's like a patient with alcohol use disorder that comes in for help and we say that maybe they'll start feeling better in three or four months. They don't want to hear that. So, this means that we have to be more aggressive and the type of probiotic selection must dramatically shift brain chemistry quickly.

For example, with alcohol use disorder, we can use high doses of bifidobacterium (up to 500 billion units daily), which helps with serotonin and dopamine regulation in the gut and the brain. And again, we aren't targeting behavior or willpower. When we correct the chemistry of the microbiome, we see dramatic results within a week or two, and then their behavior matches this improvement. They can have a dramatic reduction in alcohol cravings via shifts in the microbiome. This may seem controversial, but there is an established connection between the microbiome, the brain, and addiction. Recovery from addiction is when you rule your microbiome, and your microbiome no longer rules you.

The fascinating thing is that when you work through the gut, it can actually act like a drug, reducing alcohol cravings. People like to hear about extreme improvements and changes like this but there is some danger in it. For example, I have seen a few alcohol use disorder patients have a mild sort of serotonin syndrome from high-dose bifidobacterium due to its role in regulating gut neurotransmitter production, namely serotonin. So, we have to reduce the dosage of probiotic in these patients, and all of them were fine once we found their optimal dosage.

These kinds of microbiome shifts can result in a reduction of drug and alcohol intake, harm reduction, and improvement in nutrient status and inflammatory markers. Many of these patients also exhibit improved mood and a general increase in overall quality of life.

"It is health that is real wealth and not pieces of gold and silver."

— Mahatma Gandhi

ARE THERE SIDE EFFECTS WHEN YOU TAKE PROBIOTICS?

Absolutely! Remember that the gut regulates the bioavailability and production of neurotransmitters. So, if you take someone who's on an antidepressant, for example, and introduce them to high-dose bacteria that regulates the production of serotonin, you have to be very cautious because you can trigger side effects. This shows the ultimate potency of working through the gut. Like I mentioned before, you can get drug-like effects by manipulating the microbiome.

A potential side effect of this could be increased anxiety or aggravation of existing symptoms, such as agitation and gastrointestinal discomfort. This doesn't mean that probiotics aren't a very useful tool and shouldn't be used. You just have to be mindful of the therapeutic approach to improve these people's microbiomes that are so severely damaged. For these extreme cases, we must take our time and be gentler with the improvement of the microbiome so that their body can adjust gradually.

The other factor that comes into play is the competition of other bacteria and bugs. As you're killing off the bad bacteria, they are actually creating chemicals that support junk-food seeking behavior that feed them. So, if you're killing off and suppressing bugs that have actually been regulating your appetite, you're going to have extreme cravings, anxiety, and fatigue. Patients experience withdrawal and die-off toxicity almost to the point of saying, "Something's wrong! I should be feeling better, not worse." The feeling of frustration is compounded because you're eating healthy foods like fruits and vegetables, but you feel like you're starving.

Your body is not starving, because you're eating thousands of calories found within fruits, vegetables and lean organic protein. You're just starving off the bad bacteria and growing the good bacteria. In the example of alcohol use disorder, we wouldn't necessarily increase their cravings, because they're already addicted to alcohol. But we could increase other issues like anxiety and mood disruption. However, in these extreme cases, such as in alcohol use disorder, I don't see these severe side effects much because their microbiomes are already so disrupted that they actually recover pretty quickly.

The side effects like anxiety and mood issues generally come from the people that are unaware of their disrupted microbiome. In these people, it's a little bit subtler. I mentioned instances like this in the chapter on diet, Chapter 7. If you remove certain foods, you can create the same kind of side effects. It's not that you're making things worse, it's just that the bad bacteria are basically screaming out at you to feed them. So, while it *feels* like things are getting worse, you're actually getting better.

Another issue that this poses then is that the natural reaction or instinct would be for someone to think, "This isn't working. It's making me worse, so I shouldn't continue or keep doing this."

But the reality is that what's really making you sick is all of the junk that you've been consuming, which has destroyed your microbiome ecosystem. Once we kill off all of the imposters (bad bacteria) and increase the good bacteria, these side effects will go away. And as I mentioned before, the majority of people experience an improvement in less than the first thirty days.

SOURCES OF PROBIOTICS

Because the gut's health is determined by your diet (what you consume), at NutriChem we have microbiome nutritionists on staff to assist us in creating and designing diets, supplements, bacteria, and fibers to help patients stimulate microbiome recovery.

Below is a list of good probiotic sources that microbiome nutritionists would recommend (all are fermented):

- Kefir
- Yogurt with live active cultures
- Pickled vegetables
- Tempeh
- Kombucha tea

- Kimchi
- Miso
- Sauerkraut

BRAIN POWER TIP

When you're altering the microbiome, you could experience some of the same side effects that occur when removing an addictive drug. These side effects can be severe, but we monitor this with each patient to ensure that the recovery process is as smooth and gradual as it needs to be.

While probiotics can help stimulate recovery in the microbiome, true healing and rejuvenation stems from a healthy diet. Through your diet comes good health or poor health. The purpose of the diet, probiotics, and prebiotics is to starve and remove the harmful bacteria and restore and feed good bacteria.

And even though some may experience side effects as a direct result of the severity of their disrupted microbiome and their addiction to specific substances (drugs, food, alcohol, etc.), the majority of people experience a significant improvement in their health within the first thirty days.

(RECOMMENDATION: BRAIN POWER TIP)

If you drink alcohol, it is important to know that certain probiotics have shown to help reduce harm from alcohol consumption and cravings for alcohol. If you drink alcohol, consider using probiotics to mitigate its potentially harmful effects.

Also, people who consume alcohol can get liver cirrhosis with highly varied amounts of alcohol intake. A healthy microbiome has shown to reduce risk of liver cirrhosis in alcohol use disorder.

So, if you drink alcohol regularly, take probiotics.

CHAPTER 9

PREBIOTICS (FIBERS)

"I am an invisible man. I am a man of substance, of flesh and bone, fiber and liquids—and I might even be said to possess a mind. I am invisible, understand, simply because people refuse to see me."

— Ralph Ellison

I love this quote. While Ralph Ellison wasn't talking about the microbiome, it fits perfectly with what we've been discussing. Up until now, you've most likely been unaware of the microbiome's existence. And of the few who might have had a suspicion, you had limited information about its importance.

So, for me, I like to see it as the "invisible man" of medicine that no one knows exists because they choose not to see him. But now your eyes have been opened! And you're aware of the microbiome and its importance for your health.

We've touched on prebiotics or fibers briefly in earlier chapters, but we're going to dive deeper now. Before we continue, it's vital that you understand what prebiotics are and are not.

Prebiotics are:
- the truest, most effective source for overall health in the microbiome and brain
- proven to reduce bad cholesterol, improve heart health, improve immune system function, prevent bowel diseases, reduce inflammation, and increase lifespan
- fibers found in fruits and vegetables
- undigested by humans, but digested extensively by gut bacteria
- the fuel source for good bacteria
- a natural remedy to health problems
- the answer to having a healthy microbiome

Prebiotics are not:
- just something your grandma takes so that she can go to the bathroom

In Chapter 8, we discussed probiotics and their benefits. The only thing that you need to solidify in your memory is that probiotics are good bacteria that your microbiome requires for healthy functioning. And prebiotics are the FOOD for that good bacteria. Prebiotics are simply the fibers that feed healthy probiotic bacteria. And different prebiotic fibers can grow virtually all of the key bacterial groups in a healthy microbiome, compared to probiotics, which can only increase approximately one quarter of these bacterial groups.

Prebiotics (soluble fibers) are the fuel for the microbiome. However, with the trillion-dollar food industry pumping out processed foods, we have a health epidemic of tremendous proportions. People, especially in North America, have become accustomed to processed foods made to be cheap and convenient.

But there's a darker side to the food industry that many refuse to consider. Many of the processed foods that you consume on a daily basis are contaminated with preservatives, refined sugars, pesticides, antibiotics, and growth hormones, which negatively affect your microbiome. In addition, many of these "foods" are highly addictive because of their ability to alter gut and brain chemistry.

While people look to over one million different products to restore their health and cure their anxiety and depression, or increase their longevity, I can assure you that these gimmicky products are not the answer. Nothing has more evidence of extending your life and improving your health than soluble fiber. Soluble fiber seems to positively impact every major modern, chronic disease.

The health industry wants your attention on the millions of other products that treat symptoms, but never the root issue, because there's massive profit involved. However, the simple fact is that the answer to your health problems is something you can obtain simply through eating more fruits and vegetables, as well as asking yourself an important question: "How much soluble fiber am I eating each day?" This is a question that most people cannot answer. Even the most conservative food guides recommend 10-15 grams per day, and in my practice, I recommend at least 10-15 grams per day from NON-GRAIN sources (not wheat). Current Canadian guidelines recommend approximately 30g of total fiber daily for most adults.

Our bodies cannot digest fiber, but the good bacteria in our guts can. They love it! It's their natural food source. The unfortunate fact is that almost no one gets enough soluble fiber. It's not sexy. As I mentioned above, it's something that we typically believe old people need to take in order to use the bathroom. While this does help them have normal bowel movements, there's a deeper and more prominent reason for this and it transcends age.

Most of us are deficient in soluble fiber, but it is one of the only nutrients that has been proven to increase lifespan. There are several different types of prebiotic fibers that we commonly use at NutriChem. One such type of fiber are polyphenolics. Polyphenolics are very potent and well-tolerated, and include hesperidin and naringin, which I put in NutriChem's product *Factor 4 Fiber* when I designed it. Another important type of fiber are oligosaccharides (undigested sugars that only bacteria can digest e.g. inulin, FOS, GOS, XOS, etc.). Another type of fiber that we use are resistant starches, such as those from cooled potatoes. At the end of this chapter, I'll provide a Fiber Chart that outlines various forms of fibers, their food sources, and their benefit to your health.

Many years ago, when I was just getting started in the pharmaceutical industry, if I would give three people fiber, one would improve, one would get worse, and one would stay neutral. I wondered why that was, but now I know.

Fibers are great for maintaining healthy microbiomes but may not be appropriate to initially treat someone with a disrupted microbiome. As a general rule, fiber feeds good bacteria, but they can also feed some bad bacteria as well. This is why it's key to understand how the microbiome works and attack the root causes of disruption.

At NutriChem, we focus on the root problem when designing a customized health plan for a patient. We use a structured approach when implementing fibers to ensure their effectiveness. We often begin with gentle, well-tolerated fiber like a polyphenolic (Factor 4 Fiber) to initially start repairing the gut lining. Once we've improved the lining wall, killed off some of the nasty strains of bacteria, and shifted the gut towards healthier bacterial strains, we can use other fibers like oligosaccharides (e.g. XOS) and resistant starch to grow healthy gut bacteria in bulk.

It's worth noting here that the gut cannot tolerate this source of fuel until the microbiome's health has been improved. If we give oligosaccharide fibers to an unhealthy microbiome, bad bacteria can propagate and patients' gut symptoms can actually be exacerbated. They can get extreme gas, bloating, diarrhea, constipation, and stomach upset. We don't want these patients to think that fiber is bad for them, when it is actually ultimately the best thing for them. An unhealthy microbiome is not in the right condition to use fibers beneficially. The fibers are being used by inflammatory gas-producing bacteria that are still present in their disrupted gut. Until we've killed off most of the bad bacteria that disrupts the microbiome, we are cautious about giving oligosaccharides like inulin or XOS because we do not want to grow more of these bad bacteria.

We need to fix the microbiome through a 30-day adjusted diet, and only then lock in those changes with soluble fiber. You lock in the changes because you continue to grow and nourish healthy bacterial structures with soluble fibers. If you cease nourishing these bacteria, they deteriorate and bad bacteria eventually return.

Let's look at the *Fiber Chart* for the various types of fibers (these are soluble and insoluble fibers), their derivative source, and health benefits.

FIBER CHART

FIBER	DERIVATIVE SOURCE	HEALTH BENEFITS
Inulin	• Extracted from chicory root • A polysaccharide and fructan • Found in vegetable roots and rhizomes that do not produce starch • A FODMAP source	Helps improve mineral absorption and may help reduce triglycerides and cholesterol
Psyllium Husk Whole	• Mucinage is derived from the seed coating (husk) • Water-soluble but swells to create a gel • A polysaccharide but also has a high percentage of hemicellulose	Shown to reduce cholesterol and glucose levels; relatively resistant to fermentation
Psyllium Husk Powdered	• Powdered husk absorbs water to create a gel • Partially fermentable, but not as fermentable as the seed because of its high hemicellulose content	Provides same health benefits as non-powdered husk, but creates a smoother texture when mixed with liquid
Psyllium Seed	• Husk and seed powder combination • Also, a polysaccharide, non-starch, but more fermentable than the husk	Fermentation produces the short-chain fatty acids (SCFAs) acetate, propionate, and butyrate * Note: Taking the seed and the husk together is the most effective use. The husk brings the seed fiber further down the intestinal tract so that more fermentation takes place in the colon and less in the small intestine
Oat Fibre – β Glucan	Soluble and fermentable fiber from oats	• Oat β Glucan is a water-soluble fiber that lowers serum cholesterol • 3g / day of oat fiber can lower total cholesterol by up to 5% • Can help normalize digestive transit time
Citrus Pectin	Concentrated in the pulp and peel of citrus fruits	Studies show that it's an effective lead chelation therapy for children hospitalized for lead poisoning

FIBER	DERIVATIVE SOURCE	HEALTH BENEFITS
Modified Citrus Pectin	• Concentrated in the pulp and peel of citrus fruits • Modified = hydrolyzed.	• Shown to block cancer metastasis • Galactose in MCP binds to galectins on cancer cells, which inhibits it's adhesion to normal cells (14) Note: Studies done in breast and colon cancer patients • May chelate to heavy metals and lower cholesterol (more research is being conducted to understand this more)
Guar Gum	• Galactomannan soluble fiber made from hydrolyzed guar gum (from guar beans) • Also used in food processing as a gelling agent	• Improves mineral absorption • Helps to stabilize blood sugar • Lowers LDL cholesterol and triglycerides • Feeds healthy bacteria to increase SCFAs
Resistant Starch (RS)	• Starch that functions as a dietary fiber • Several different types found in many plant-based foods (e.g. nuts, seeds, legumes, potatoes, plantains, bananas, etc.) • Starches higher in amylose • Whole food starches naturally have some resistant starch present • If the starch is turned into flour (e.g. wheat flour), resistant starch will be lowered • However, cooking increases resistant starch content via retrogradation	4 types: RS1: Found in nuts, seeds, and legumes. RS2: Starch that is inaccessible to enzymes due to its high amylose content. Examples: raw green bananas, plantains, and raw potato. RS3: Formed by retrogradation. Note: Similar to gelatinization. RS3 is formed by cooking and cooling a starchy food. For example, cooled potato starch RS4: Modified in a lab to resist digestion. Feeds bacteria to produce butyrate, propionate, and acetate.
FOS – Fructooligosaccharides Or oligofructan	• Used as a prebiotic in several supplements • Naturally found in foods like onion, garlic, chicory, artichoke, and asparagus	• Metabolized by intestinal flora to form short-chain carboxylic acids, L-lactate, and CO2 • Shown to improve mineral absorption and decrease serum cholesterol levels
GOS – galactooligosaccha-rides or oligolactose	• Produced through enzyme conversion of lactose • Used as a prebiotic in infant formulas	• Used in constipation relief Note: Studied in infants and elderly.

151

FIBER	DERIVATIVE SOURCE	HEALTH BENEFITS
XOS – xylooligosaccharide	• XOS are sugar oligomers made up of xylose units, which appear in bamboo shoots, fruits, vegetables, milk, and honey • Supplements are produced in a lab from lignocellulosic materials (LCMs)	• Study found it to increase bifidobacterium count without increasing lactobacillus • Reduces fat production in the liver • Increases cholesterol excretion • Acts as a dietary fiber • Shown to feed mainly bifido strains of bacteria without feeding pathogenic ("bad bacteria") strains
PGX	• Patented water-soluble polysaccharide complex	• Shown to lower LDL and total cholesterol • Used before meals as an appetite suppressant and blood sugar stabilizer • Feeds good bacteria, which increases SCFAs
Larch arabinogalactan	• Highly branched polysaccharide from larch tree (a deciduous conifer)	• Feeds lactobacillus and bifidobacterium • Increases SCFAs and decreases absorption and production of ammonia • Can help with certain cancer treatments because it has been shown to stimulate Natural Killer cells and prevent metastasis to the liver • May help with chronic viral infections.
Polyphenolic Fibers	• Citrus fruits, citrus fruit peels, grapes, wine	• Grow healthy bacterial groups Clostridia Clusters IV and XIV • Have shown to help weight loss and improve blood sugar levels • Natural antioxidants • Help to repair the digestive tract lining

BRAIN POWER TIP

Prebiotics (soluble fiber) are a great source of improved and lasting health, but not the solution to a damaged microbiome.

Before fibers can effectively maintain your health, you must fix the microbiome by eradicating the bad bacteria found within.

You do this via a modified diet, such as a paleo diet or FODMAP diet. This starves out the bad bacteria to enable new growth for good bacteria. Then, when fiber is introduced and continued, the good bacteria thrive and build up a protective shield to resist and prevent bad (harmful) bacteria from infiltrating the microbiome in the future.

Probiotics (good bacteria) and prebiotics (soluble fiber) work hand-in-hand to kill off bad bacteria and restore microbiome health. For temporary relief from symptoms, taking fiber will improve your "symptoms" of poor health, but will be rendered ineffective long-term without correcting the microbiome first.

We'll discuss *Microbiotic Manipulation* in the next chapter.

THE REAL TIP:
Probiotics are great, but soluble fiber will grow more probiotic bacteria than taking any probiotic product.

"When your body absorbs toxins, it stores them in fat, which is why fiber and probiotics are strategic weapons for weight loss. Fiber keeps your colon healthy and reduces your body's absorption of toxins."

— Suzanne Somers

CHAPTER 10

MICROBIOTIC MANIPULATION

"In the future, every pharmacist should know what a given drug does to the microbiome."

– Kent MacLeod

This chapter is about the 50% of people that do not get a full response to our microbiome treatment plans within the first 30 days. We'll cover how:

- Not everyone responds to diet, probiotics, and prebiotics.
- There are bacteria and fungi that must be killed off, and are difficult to kill off, before certain people can shift their microbiome effectively.
- There are certain herbal antimicrobials that have proven to be as effective as many antibiotics for killing biofilm-forming microorganisms.
- There are other herbals, with less scientific evidence, that have been used traditionally to treat gastrointestinal issues.

We are beginning to realize that almost all substances, be it a drug, a food, or a drink, impact the microbiome, and we must be aware of this. RESPECT THE MICROBIOME! DISRESPECT IT AT YOUR PERIL!

For certain patients, we have to dig deeper into their issues with specific testing. Using urinary organic acid testing (a urine sample), we can look at signs of bacterial or fungal overgrowth and biofilms that may not be treatable with diet, probiotics, and prebiotics. We also look at stool samples for bacterial strains, and perform bacterial DNA testing to identify what bugs are currently residing in your gut.

We are just now beginning to awaken to the fact that any time that you change your diet, fibers, drugs, or herbs, you are always shifting or manipulating the microbiome. Anything that you intake, be it food, drink, or drugs, can impact the microbiome. Exercise, sleep, and stress reduction have also shown to improve the health of the microbiome.

An interesting example is the drug, metformin. Metformin has been the number one oral drug used to treat Type 2 diabetes for decades. Initially, we thought that this drug sensitized the body to insulin via the pancreas or liver, but recent studies have shown that metformin actually exerts its effects via the microbiome.

Just as with metformin, we assume that a drug has a specific benefit on the body by binding specific receptors. However, many of these drugs are actually impacting the microbiome, which then has a widespread effect on the rest of the body and brain.

Another drug example that I mentioned in Chapter 2 is proton pump inhibitors, or PPIs. PPIs were believed to have virtually no negative impact on the body, but we now know that over time, these drugs can cause several harmful side effects. The rule I stress with patients is, "Do not take anything unless you know its impact on the microbiome first."

As a pharmacist, I think that all healthcare providers should be held responsible for knowing all of the side effects of consuming any pharmaceutical drug, food, or drink, and this includes the impact on the microbiome. You are not really doing your job as a pharmacist if you do not know how a given drug impacts the microbiome.

Whether it's a seemingly innocent soft drink or an insidious illegal narcotic, pharmacists should understand how these chemicals impact the gut once ingested. For example, we know that the sugar in soft drinks is bad for the microbiome. When we began to recognize the negative health impact of sugar, diet soft drinks were created. But it's now been proven that the artificial sweeteners contained in these diet soft drinks are also very damaging to the microbiome, despite having less calories.

In the future, as the pharmaceutical industry catches up to this realization, a well-informed pharmacist will always assess a drug's impact on the microbiome, as well as evaluate other safety precautions. In addition, they will recommend precision-dosed, individualized supplements (e.g. multivitamins, fibers, diets, etc.) specific to each patient's needs.

Healthcare will hopefully become more aware of the importance of the microbiome, and treatments will become far more individualized and precise depending on each patient's unique needs.

THE PROCESS OF CHANGE

Changing the microbiome is actually an easy feat in theory, but it requires diligent effort on the patient's part. It isn't necessarily easy to do psychologically, because you have to break bad dietary habits and mindsets. But in some cases, it can be very difficult because certain people do not respond to our diets, probiotics, and fibers. We see these non-responders more and more frequently. So, what about the resistant cases?

The diet, probiotics, and fibers that we have can make big shifts in the majority of people's microbiomes alone. But some individuals come to us with resistant gastrointestinal bacteria and fungi that cause very serious health issues. The microorganisms can form highly resistant films, called *biofilms*. Antibiotics cannot penetrate them, and people end up with resistant infections and colonizations of bad bacteria and fungi in these biofilms.

These biofilms impede good bacteria from rooting in the gut. Most disease-causing bacteria actually form these biofilms, and antibiotics and healthy bacteria cannot get past the biofilm barrier. If antibiotics cannot penetrate these, we have to start looking to natural herbals and other remedies to try to kill off bad, biofilm-producing bacteria and fungi.

There are many natural herbals that act as antimicrobials and biofilm busters, and they are actually more effective than most antibiotics. An example is the bismuth nitrate molecules. These have shown in many studies to be more effective than many antibiotics for treating gut infections that form biofilms. These include herbals, bismuth nitrates (alone or in combination with different thiols), berberine, oregano oil, garlic, frankincense, myrrh, black cumin seed oil, and caprylic acid. There are many conditions that are untreatable with antibiotics, so we have to use natural antimicrobials in some cases. I have treated many patients that have become very resistant to antibiotics, but often they will have good responses to herbal antimicrobial therapy.

I had a 30-year-old male come to my office one day complaining of alcoholism, alcoholic neuropathy, depression, and anxiety.

He had been drinking nine or more drinks every day for the last nine years. He was taking multiple medications for his health problems:
Gabapentin 3600 mg for his alcoholic neuropathy.
Wellbutrin 100mg for his severe depression.

Trazodone 100mg for his insomnia.

He also took multivitamins, benfotiamine, vitamin B6 (not P5P), and vitamin B12.

He complained about severe indigestion, burping, bloating, cramping, alternating diarrhea and constipation, and had a history of severe digestive problems that had lasted for as long as he could remember. These only worsened over time as his alcohol intake increased.

I found it odd that he didn't even mention his digestive problems as a primary complaint. I had to dig this out of him as he elaborated upon different symptoms. After we performed our Full-body Chemistry Test, the lab showed that he had a functional B12 deficiency, low testosterone, and other nutrient deficiencies. According to the Beck Depression Inventory, his score was 48, which correlates to extreme depression.

My assessment of his health was severe digestion problems as a direct result of a disrupted microbiome, which was contributing to his poor quality of life, addiction, anxiety, and depression.

The plan-of-attack that I implemented for this young man was a 30-day modified paleo diet with the following additional supplements:

- GI rescue with gut-healing zinc carnosine, aloe vera, n-acetyl-glucosamine, and glutamine
- High-dose probiotics — 300 billion CFU (*Bifidobacterium longum, S. Boulardii*)
- Inulin fiber
- Customized multivitamins
- Magnesium glycinate

Within thirty days, he experienced a 70% resolution of gastrointestinal issues. He had a complete resolution of his neuropathy. His gabapentin intake had been reduced by 50% of the original dose. He had a 90% reduction of alcohol consumption with the *Bifidobacterium* probiotics. He currently reports total abstinence. He discontinued his Wellbutrin and his Beck Depression Inventory score was reduced to 16, 3 months later, which correlates to only a mild mood disturbance.

As you can see, by merely adjusting his diet and a few key supplements, we were able to resolve over 70% of his health problems. His current ongoing plan is to continue taking the vitamins, fiber, and magnesium, and to refer to the NutriChem nutrition team on an as-needed basis. He is working towards a complete resolution of all digestive problems as he maintains his doses of fiber and probiotics.

HOW DO YOU TREAT PATIENTS WHO DO NOT RESPOND TO INITIAL THERAPIES?

Microbiome Manipulation is the use of antimicrobial herbs and "biofilm busters" to shift the microbiome even more rapidly than simply using diet, probiotics, and/or prebiotics. We do this by using natural antimicrobials to kill off bad bacteria while simultaneously increasing good bacteria. It's important to remember that problematic inflammatory bacteria and fungi cause the cravings or the feeling of "starving" that patients experience during their microbiome reboot.

This is generally ascribed to willpower or the need for a reward due to the addiction of junk food or sugars from sweets, but bad bacteria and fungi love sugar. They influence your brain's cravings through the gut to maintain sugar addiction to try to ensure their own survival. With severe cases of poor diet, we need to accelerate the response.

Most extreme cases with side effects happen because people are hooked on junk food, and when these foods are removed, they have a bad reaction to the bacterial die-off effect. On average, this reaction lasts one to two weeks. During this time, however, they feel as though they need this crappy food in order to feel better. The truth is, their microbiome is severely imbalanced due to the shifting and manipulation that the junk food has had on them.

During this die-off phase, we are shifting the levels of bad and good bacteria. As we kill off the bad bacteria, the body goes into a sort of shock. But in reality, the body is fine and actually improving. The real issue of why the body feels like it's starving is because the bad bacteria and fungi are dying and they're trying to convince the brain to feed them the junk food that they crave.

As I mentioned, this typically lasts less than two weeks. Once the bad bacteria are gone, the side effects and cravings go with them.

BRAIN POWER TIP

If you have complex issues, such as anxiety, depression, fibromyalgia, chronic pain, etc., let us help you!

If you're unable to visit us here in Ottawa, Canada, then I strongly advise you visit your doctor and have them run tests on your stool, urine, and blood, then send them our way so we can properly assess your microbiome's health and prescribe you the right and most effective dietary plan to achieve optimal health.

CHAPTER 11

MENTAL HEALTH

"The most challenging epidemics
in modern society are connected
to lifestyle, and lifestyle is how
we "talk" to our microbiome."

– Deepak Chopra

We're currently seeing an epidemic of mental health disorders. These include conditions that affect both the young and the old, including anxiety, depression, addiction, Alzheimer's dementia, Parkinson's disease, ADHD, chronic pain disorders (e.g. fibromyalgia), and more. Studies have shown that almost all of these mental health conditions have a strong connection to disruptions in the microbiome.

These disorders lead to a variety of direct and indirect losses. The most common is the loss of quality of life. These deficits then impact family and friends and those involved with the care of these people. The cost of mental health disorders to society is staggering. The Canadian government estimates that the cost of mental health in Canada alone will increase to 2.3 trillion dollars by 2030.

Still, the medical industry spends billions annually on medications that don't work very well. For example, drugs used to treat Alzheimer's aim to increase the levels of acetylcholine in the brain, but they are not even modestly effective. I sympathize with the physicians who want to help their patients and it's impressive that we're able to design these drugs to try to help people, but the problem is that they simply aren't working.

From my experience, when we use many of these drugs to treat certain mental health conditions, we are just treating surface symptoms, not the root cause. Throughout my career, I have seen many categories of ineffective or inappropriate psychiatric drugs used in these patients, including antidepressants, benzodiazepines, cholinesterase inhibitors, and opioids. In my clinical practice, there are many mental health conditions that actually respond quite well to microbiome and lifestyle treatments, such as anxiety, mild to moderate depression, addictions, chronic pain conditions (e.g. fibromyalgia), chronic fatigue, ADHD, Alzheimer's, and even autism. Our results are more consistent in some of these areas than others, but microbiome treatments are always safe and effective. In other conditions, such as schizophrenia, bipolar disorder, Parkinson's Disease, and severe depression, there are definite links to the microbiome, but drugs are often required to help manage their symptoms while working on their gut health. Drugs are important tools in these patients, and in these complex psychiatric conditions, we often require symptomatic management with drugs while we work on underlying biochemical issues, such as microbiome status, nutrient levels, and hormone balance.

When the psychiatric drug industry is worth a trillion dollars, you know something must be off balance. If we truly want to solve the mental health crisis, we must dig deeper into what is actually happening within the body and brain. This leads to an emerging understanding and study of neuroinflammation. For example, we now know that in conditions like Alzheimer's and Parkinson's Disease, inflammation of the brain plays a major role in disease development. And as we've discussed in the previous chapters, many of the health problems that afflict millions around the world are a direct result of inflammation, and a compromised microbiome is often the main source of full-body and brain inflammation. Research is now pointing to the concept that many mental health conditions, in general, are related to brain and nervous system inflammation.

Of course, there are also very important psychological issues, such as early-life experience, that affect the development and chemistry of the brain. But I would argue that the microbiome is just as important as childhood experience on the brain's development. Poor childhood diet and nutritional neglect are forms of early childhood trauma that can powerfully affect brain chemistry. Adverse childhood experiences definitely affect the biology of the brain, but so does the microbiome! Now don't get me wrong- I don't think you are abusing or neglecting your child if you don't feed them some amazing diet. But I do wish that parents were more aware that feeding children a poor diet can negatively impact their brains.

I have been skeptical of drugs for many years, but let's say that we do ascribe to the theory that many of these mental health conditions are related to low levels of specific biochemicals in the brain, such as low acetylcholine in Alzheimer's, or low serotonin in anxiety and depression. An analogy I often use to describe the difference between what a drug does and what the microbiome and nutrients do is that many of these drugs act sort of like taps on a faucet. A drug can only increase the flow of the "water" (e.g. neurotransmitter) that is available, whereas nutrients can actually increase the amount of total "water" (neurotransmitter) that will be available. For example, an SSRI antidepressant can only increase the flow of already-available serotonin into synapses in the brain, whereas the nutrients, tryptophan or 5-HTP, can actually increase the total serotonin available at brain synapses. It is safer and more effective to increase total serotonin at these synapses with a nutrient than it is to "squeeze" a little more serotonin into the synapses with a drug.

ALZHEIMER'S, CHOLINE, AND THE MICROBIOME

It's fascinating that the sector of the pharmaceutical industry focused on Alzheimer's designs drugs that try to increase acetylcholine in the brain. Meanwhile, 95% of the world's population is deficient in choline. Most of us, including scientists, don't even know anything about choline metabolism, absorption, or function in the brain. Billions are spent on drugs every year to improve choline and acetylcholine status in elderly people. These people are typically missing choline from their diets. Most of the choline that we need comes from egg yolks or organ meats like liver. An interesting side note is the debate for the anti-cholesterol industry that says egg yolks are bad for you.

The truth is that egg yolks are the best source of choline you can find! This fact becomes even more interesting as we dive deeper into choline and the microbiome.

The bioavailability of choline is dependent on a healthy microbiome. If your microbiome is damaged, you could convert choline into inflammatory compounds that can actually harm the body. This becomes interesting when you see, for example, someone on the Mediterranean diet, which positively influences brain and heart health. This diet has a lot of choline in it compared to other diets, but it is considered "heart-healthy" because it is also a microbiome-healthy diet. Giving choline with a poor diet or an unhealthy microbiome, however, can actually lead to inflammation and may lead to an increased risk of heart attack and stroke. So, we need a knowledge of choline metabolism and the microbiome's role in this metabolism to effectively use choline.

The ironic and disappointing thing is that we have a billion-dollar industry that focuses on choline, but no one is actively telling people how to use it or get it into their brains. And that's just one nutrient that is influenced and affected by the microbiome. There are many other nutrients affected and influenced by the microbiome.

LINKING BLOOD SUGAR (DIABETES) AND ALZHEIMER'S

There was a recent research study that proved that blood sugar levels inversely correlate to cognition. What does that mean? To say it in layman's terms: "The higher your blood sugar levels are, the dumber you become." And what I mean by "dumber" is the inability to think, focus, concentrate, and perform other cognitive tasks. As blood sugar levels rise beyond the normal range, your thinking becomes less efficient.

As one could conclude from this correlation, if we have a landslide of diabetes cases, then we should also expect a landslide of cognitive disease cases, like Alzheimer's dementia, to follow. The main reason for this epidemic is because sugar is a very inflammatory substance to the gut and the brain. High blood sugar levels inflame the brain.

And what's the most powerful way to regulate one's blood sugar? The answer: the microbiome. And guess what? High blood sugar levels trigger more sugar cravings via the microbiome, and, in turn, you eat more sugar and drive up your blood sugar. You become stuck in a vicious cycle of high blood sugar and sugar cravings due to a disrupted microbiome. Some of the nastiest bacteria and fungi absolutely love to eat sugar!

In fact, the most effective drug used to treat Type 2 diabetes is called metformin. And invariably, one of its most vital benefits is improving someone's microbiome. Recent studies have shown that metformin's effects very likely occur through a microbiome mechanism.

What this means is that if we're going to truly discuss cognitive function, we need to understand how to regulate blood sugar levels through the microbiome.

Oh, and by the way, the drugs that we have discussed many times in this book, known as the proton pump inhibitors, have been strongly linked to Alzheimer's as well. Shifting the microbiome can have a profound effect on the brain and cognition!

ANTIDEPRESSANTS AND SSRIS: ANXIETY AND DEPRESSION

Another drug target example (like choline) are SSRIs (Selective Serotonin Reuptake Inhibitors). These are a psychiatric favorite. They're given to many people with various forms of anxiety and depression. SSRIs have been shown to cause cognitive impairment in many of the patients who take them. And yet, the medical industry prescribes these medications too often, without even fully understanding serotonin metabolism itself.

Serotonin regulation comes from the gut as does the bioavailability of serotonin in the brain. The main issue that I have with these drugs are that they have been shown in large studies and meta-analyses to be no better than a placebo in mild to moderate depression, but they have many serious side effects, such as weight gain, sleep disturbances, mood shifts, and sexual dysfunction. Some studies have even shown that several of these antidepressant medications are actually associated with an increased risk of suicide in certain patients.

The real problem stems from ignorance. We have this billion-dollar industry dealing with serotonin, yet, we don't even consider how important the microbiome is for serotonin production and availability for the brain. We know that the majority of serotonin is made in the gut, and that serotonin production is also dependent on certain key nutrients, such as vitamin B6 and tryptophan. Yet, we would rather give SSRIs than any of these other options.

As a pharmacologist myself with over thirty-five years' experience in the industry, if I have a pharmacological target, why wouldn't I understand the target? For example, if serotonin is the target, then a pharmacist should understand and know that the microbiome is connected and responsible for the effective production and regulation of serotonin in the body and the brain. In addition, they should understand the microbiome's activation of vitamin B6 and other nutrients involved in tryptophan and serotonin synthesis.

The same thing happens with Alzheimer's disease and other cognitive impairments or deficiencies. If you believe that acetylcholine is the target in Alzheimer's, then you have to be aware of how acetylcholine is synthesized and metabolized in the brain. Likewise, if you believe that serotonin is the ultimate target in anxiety and depression, then you have to be aware of how serotonin is metabolized in the brain as well. There are many classes of drugs like this- where the drug tries to tinker with a level of a given metabolite or neurotransmitter but ignores the actual natural source of the chemical itself. This goes back to my "drug as a mere faucet" analogy.

In conclusion, it is ironic that these natural treatments that are safe and effective are often dismissed, yet we rely on medications that are proven to be ineffective and harmful. In some cases, drugs can be very helpful, especially in very severe cases of mental illness, but why are they first-line options in all of these conditions? Although I am a pharmacist, I do not agree with putting all of these patients on drugs without even considering these other options.

THE DEVELOPING BRAIN

Today, we are seeing more and more children who suffer from behavioral or cognitive disorders. And as these numbers grow, so do the number of medications being prescribed to treat these conditions.

The sad truth is that more children are being diagnosed with attention deficit disorders. The question we should ask ourselves is *why*. We're quick to label and prescribe, but slow to understand the real nature of what's happening to our children.

They are treated with stimulant drugs that have significant adverse effects. They can produce results very quickly, but the long-term side effects on the brain are unknown. I acknowledge that for some kids, this can be the difference between academic success or failure, but at what cost? No matter how we spin it, we are giving children very powerful stimulants and amphetamines.

Meanwhile, there are proven links between the disruption of the gut, and cognitive function, focus issues, and brain development. Bottom line is, if you don't have a healthy microbiome, your brain will not develop correctly.

I have one patient who's a third-grade teacher. She told me that at least one-third of her class suffers from *severe* mental or behavioral health problems. Imagine how difficult it is for someone to manage those kids, much less educate them? And then what about the impact on the education and learning of the other two-thirds of the class? Many schools have classes full of kids with behavioral and mental health problems, but we can't just medicate these issues away. No parent wants to medicate their child, but these drugs are the first-line option for all of these kids with almost no consideration for the digestive tract's role in their behavior. What if we just started treating these children's digestive problems and examined how much that helped their behavior? In my experience, doing this has dramatic effects that are more impressive than any drug.

BRAIN POWER TIP

Exercise!
Do you struggle with your mood?

Did you know that exercise has been proven to be as effective as antidepressants for anxiety and mild to moderate depression?

And even better, studies have shown that exercise improves microbiome health by shifting gut bacteria towards increased growth of beneficial bacterial strains.

So, if you want to boost your microbiome and your mood, get moving! Just 30-60 minutes of moderate exercise, especially cardiovascular exercise, can help combat gastrointestinal issues, as well as anxiety and depression!

Only you can decide, but I'm here to help you get your life back. Let me show you how.

"I'm a big believer that life changes as much as you want it to."

— Martin Freeman

CHAPTER 12

CASE STUDIES

"To become an academic expert takes
years of studying. Academic experts
are experts in how and what others
have done. They use case studies and
observation to understand a subject."

— Simon Sinek

In this final chapter, I want to illustrate through "proof-of-evidence" that what I've shared with you in this book is not science fiction or fantasy. It is real and very possible in your life today.

What you will read are case studies from patients, just like you, who suffered from a wide variety of mental and physical illnesses.

CASE #1 — DOWN SYNDROME, MICROBIOME, AND SEIZURES

Review of Systems/Background:
- 25-year-old female (American)
- Down Syndrome (Trisomy 21)
- Always had problems with stomach upset, constipation
- Had seizures frequently (3 seizures per week)

I avoid giving "standard" fibers (e.g. Metamucil, inulin) to people with stomach problems because many of these fibers could create bad side effects. If they already have a disrupted microbiome, this could make the problem worse. Giving "standard fiber" to people with GI problems could have varied and seemingly random effects.

People with Down Syndrome have been shown in studies to have lower nutrient levels, which, over time, could impact the microbiome.

Allergies/Sensitivities:
- No known drug or food allergies
- Gluten sensitivity (on a gluten-free diet)

Medical History:
- Down Syndrome
- Epilepsy
- Multiple Knee Surgeries
- OCD (Obsessive-Compulsive Disorder)

Medications & Supplements:
- Ogestrel (Ethynyl Estradiol and Norgestrel) once daily
- Vimpat (Lacosamide) 150mg twice daily
- Keppra (Levetiracetam) 1000mg twice daily
- Rhodiola Rosea 170mg once daily

- Vitamin D3 2000IU per day
- Acetyl-L Carnitine 1000mg twice daily
- Digestive Enzymes with each meal 3 times per day
- Triphala (Herbal Blend) 250mg once daily
- Fish Oil 2 teaspoons daily
- Magnesium Glycinate 200mg twice daily
- Probiotic 50 Billion Units per day

Treatment:
- Gut Makeover Diet x 30 days
- Prebiotic Fibers (Factor 4 Fiber and Gastro Guard) twice daily
- 5-strain *Bifidobacterium* probiotic x 100B units daily

Follow-up (3 months):
- Full resolution of all constipation & stomach problems
- Seizures stopped after two months (1 incidence of dizziness, but no more seizures)
- Improvement in brain inflammation and overall inflammation (C-Reactive Protein decreased significantly)
- Improvement in cognitive function

We know that brain inflammation is affected by the gut, and this is a quintessential gut-brain connection case.

Summary:
I corresponded with the mother of the patient, not the patient directly. The patient had previously tried several anti-seizure medications, with minimal long-term benefit. I fully immersed her into my clinical practice of microbiome protocols.

The patient had seen some improvements with custom vitamin formulas—custom nutrients for Down Syndrome. However, our recent microbiome protocols had the most profound effects.

I encouraged her to continue taking her seizure medication,

levetiracetam. Due to improving her gut health, the medication began to work more efficiently and effectively. Many drugs work better when someone's gut health improves. Often, I will say, tongue-in-cheek, "You see, your medication is working better now." In reality, the drugs were not actually all that effective, but conventional medicine would claim that the drugs were responsible even though what we really changed was the microbiome.

CASE #2 — MICROBIOME, THYROID FUNCTION, AND TESTOSTERONE LEVELS IN MEN

Review of Systems/Background:
- 46-year-old male
- Consistent Hypothyroid for several years, very volatile thyroid function
- Low testosterone
- On Synthroid for thyroid replacement for 5+ years
- His doctor frequently altered his thyroid dosages for two years
- Disturbances in his metabolomics (gut disruptions & chronic stress)
- Alternating diarrhea & constipation

Microbiome disruption makes a big difference in response to thyroid replacement medications. In an unhealthy gut, a small dose change in a medication like Synthroid (levothyroxine) can result in large shifts in thyroid hormones (TSH, T3, and T4).

At first, I wondered if this man's health problems were due to a disrupted microbiome or an iodine deficiency, because we know that the microbiome affects T4 to T3 conversion. In addition, we know that some people respond to T3 (liiothyronine) but not T4 (levothyroxine).

My assessment was that the microbiome's role in converting T4 to T3 is the indicating factor. A disrupted microbiome is inefficient at converting T4 to T3. I also addressed his testosterone levels because we know that the microbiome affects both estrogen and testosterone levels. I knew that adjusting the microbiome would help with both his thyroid function and testosterone levels. We have a thyroid disfunction epidemic and a low testosterone epidemic in men. Is this due to some mysterious toxicity? No, it is due to an epidemic of poor microbiome health.

Allergies/Sensitivities:
No known allergies

Medical History:
- Hypothyroidism
- IgA Nephropathy (Berger's disease)
- Detached Retina in both eyes (surgery for both eyes)
- Low Testosterone (7-11 nmol/L range)

Medications & Supplements:
- Synthroid 100mcg daily
- AndroGel 1%- 50mg once daily (1 sachet daily)
- Fish Oil 1-2 tsp daily
- Probiotic
- Custom Multi-Vitamin Formula

Treatment:
- Gut Makeover Diet (30-Day)
- Prebiotics (Factor 4 Fibre) x 1 capsule daily
- Probiotics (S. Boulardii & Bifidobacteria Longum strains)- 50B units daily
- Microbiome modifiers (Natural antimicrobials to eliminate unhealthy gut bacteria and fungus)- Candibactin AR two tablets twice daily + Candibactin BR two tablets twice daily

Follow-up (3 months)

- Thyroid response became much more stable after microbiome protocols
- Testosterone levels shifted up to ~20nmol/L on average
- Patient felt better in general—more energy, improved libido
- Lost five pounds of fat
- Gained muscle mass
- Resolution of diarrhea & constipation

Summary:

This patient's health problems clearly illustrate the connection between the microbiome and thyroid function. When his microbiome improved, his thyroid function normalized, and his low testosterone levels increased.

The patient also lost weight, while adding muscle. This reveals the interconnection of not only the gut-thyroid relationship, but the gut with other systems of the body (i.e. endocrine function and testosterone).

Everything is interconnected.

The microbiome is the "central router" of the entire body. When it improves, other organ systems, hormone levels, and general health improves.

CASE #3 — GUT-HEART CONNECTION

Review of Systems/Background:

- 67-year-old female
- Chronic *C. Difficile* infection
- Many rounds of various antibiotics for *C. Difficile*
- Lifelong cardiovascular health problems
- GI problems—very frequent diarrhea, upset stomach
- Previous stroke, put on anticoagulant medications post-stroke (target INR= 3-4)
- INR (she was on Coumadin) was very volatile (could not get in target range of 3-4)
- On *Weight Watchers* diet

Allergies/Sensitivities:
No known allergies

Medical History:
- Previous Stroke
- Heart Palpitations
- Multiple Blood Clots after heart valve surgery (had titanium valve put in in 2003)
- Hysterectomy
- Chronic *C. difficile* Infection (multiple rounds of antibiotics)
- GI problems (upset stomach & diarrhea)

Medications & Supplements:
- 81mg ASA once daily
- 4mg warfarin once daily
- 5mg bisoprolol once daily
- Crestor 20mg once daily
- EstroGel 0.06%- apply 1 pump once daily
- Progesterone 100mg by mouth once daily at bedtime

Treatment:
- Candibactin BR 1 tablet twice daily
- Xylooligosaccharide (XOS) Factor 1 capsule daily, increased to 3
- 50 Billion units per cap multi-strain probiotic once daily
- Reduction of processed foods (patient was not ready to comply with our diet plan)
- Mega Marine 2 gel caps daily
- Mega Mag 200mg 2 caps daily
- Custom Multi-Vitamin Formula daily
- Adjustment of estrogen and progesterone dosing
- Continue *Weight Watchers Diet*

Follow-up (30 days):
- Stabilization of INR in 3-4 range, consistently
- Resolution of heart palpitations
- Improvement of diarrhea & frequent upset stomach

Summary:
This illustrates the gut-heart connection via blood coagulation and palpitations.

When we stabilized her microbiome, her coagulation status stabilized (INR stayed in more consistent 3-4 range) and her heart palpitations stopped.

More and more studies are showing that there is a relationship between gut bacterial strains and heart health, obesity, cholesterol levels, high blood pressure, atrial fibrillation, insulin resistance, inflammation, and TMAO production (a cardiotoxic metabolite that forms from choline when the gut is disrupted and certain "bad" bacteria are present in the GI tract).

CASE #4 — GUT-BRAIN CONNECTION

Review of System/Backgrounds:
- 54-year-old female
- Menopausal
- Central Sensitivity & Pain Syndrome
- Fibromyalgia
- Frequent Migraines
- Restless Leg Syndrome
- Depression
- Daily cannabis usage for pain and sleep
- Low thyroid
- Irritable Bowel Syndrome

This patient believed that one's interpretation of the world could create depression. However, I told her that a disrupted gut could cause depression, not just her perceptions of the world.

The gut-brain connection affects one's mental health and interpretation of the world. There is gut chemistry underlying mood and one's outlook of the world.

She was a good candidate for hormone treatments, however, we began treating her microbiome and thyroid first because we did not want to give hormones before we corrected her microbiome. If you don't treat the microbiome first, people don't respond as well to bio-identical hormones.

You can see unpredictable responses and the dosages required then become volatile.

Allergies/Sensitivities:
- No known allergies
- Sensitivity to dairy, gluten, etc. (Irritable Bowel Syndrome)
- Severe seasonal allergies (very reactive to pollen, mold, changes in seasons)

Medical History:
- Fibromyalgia & Chronic Pain
- Depression
- Chronic Migraines
- Hypothyroidism
- Osteoarthritis
- Menopausal symptoms (hot flashes, bloating, mood swings)
- Irritable Bowel Syndrome (IBS)
- Post-traumatic Stress Disorder
- Frequent Seasonal Allergies
- Obsessive-Compulsive Disorder (OCD)

Medications & Supplements:
- Cymbalta (duloxetine) 60mg every other day
- Advair Inhaler 2 puffs, twice daily
- Eletriptan 40mg, as needed for migraines
- Omnaris nasal spray 1-2 sprays in each nostril daily

- Multi-Vitamin once daily
- Magnesium Glycinate 825mg, twice daily (powder)
- Glucosamine/chondroitin 500/400mg, once daily
- Medical cannabis daily

Treatment:
- Gut Makeover Diet (30 Day)
- Candida Stop (had organic acid lab markers of fungal overgrowth—elevated oxalic acid)
- Probiotics (S. Boulardii & Bifidobacteria Longum strains) 1-2 caps daily (gradually increased to 3-4 times daily)
- Tyro-Trypt (5-HTP/L-Tyrosine/Vitamin B6) for mood (low dosage due to interaction with antidepressant medication)
- Deprescribing antidepressants (Cymbalta)—slow tapering regimen over 1 month as dosage of Tyro-Trypt gradually increased (a "cross-taper" with Tyro-Trypt)
- Mega Mag 200mg 1 capsule at bedtime
- Fish Oil 1 teaspoon daily with food
- Phosphogabamine (GABA, Suntheanine, Phosphatidylserine, Glutamine) 2 caps x 3 times daily for anxiety
- ND on NutriChem team prescribed Desiccated Thyroid- 30mg once daily

Follow-up (3 months):
- Significant improvement in mood (Beck Depression inventory improved from 35= "Severe" depression to 25 = "Moderate" Depression
- Symptoms of IBS improved significantly (less bloating, less nausea)
- Thyroid levels normalized
- Fibromyalgia pain significantly improved from 7/10 to 5/10 (a big difference for this patient, who had tremendous levels of persistent pain)

Summary:
This is a classic comorbid case of a patient with IBS, fibromyalgia, depression, and other mental health issues, that can link everything back to a disrupted microbiome as the cause for the full-body imbalance.

I see these sorts of gut-brain connection cases every day. I see a disproportionate number of fibromyalgia patients like this every day, if you look for them. Everyone would see this combination of conditions, if they looked for them. Nearly all of them have disrupted guts as well as anxiety and depression.

CASE #5 — RESISTANCE TO MAINTAINING MICROBIOME PROTOCOLS DESPITE IRREFUTABLE EFFECTIVENESS

Review of Systems/Background:
- 76-year-old woman
- Previous colon cancer
- Diverticulitis
- Chronic diarrhea for several years
- Osteoarthritis
- Previous hip replacement surgery
- Colorectal cancer

Treatment:
- Anti-inflammatory Diet (30 days)

We placed an emphasis on no gluten because gluten appeared to grossly trigger her inflammation and diarrhea.

- S. Boulardii probiotic 1-2 capsules daily
- Switched to 50-billion-unit multi-strain probiotic
- Candibactin BR 2 caps daily
- Factor 4 Fibre (Hesperidin and Naringin polyphenols) once daily
- Curcumin (high-dose)- BCM95 curcumin 1-2 caps daily
- Fish Oil 1-2 teaspoons daily
- Custom vitamin formula daily
- Reduce and eventually discontinue loperamide for diarrhea

Follow-up (30 days):
- Minimal diarrhea
- Significant improvement in upset stomach & symptoms of diverticulitis
- She was very surprised at how effective these protocols were toward improving her health

Summary:
She was very resistant to continue the microbiome protocols. She would say, "Now can I eat whatever I want? Do I have to keep taking the probiotic and fiber?"

It was hard to get her to continue taking fiber and probiotics, even with her history of colon cancer and diverticulitis. I would often ask her, "What is the down side to continuing to take the fiber and probiotics? It's cheap and, what's more, that's all you need to take to continue to feel better!"

Despite her new awareness of how certain foods irritated her gut, she was still resistant. Her extreme hesitation to go back to the way things were was like an alcoholic asking, "Can I go back to drinking now?" It's lunacy! But I see it all the time.

If this is still how someone thinks, then we haven't sorted out all the chemical issues yet. She eventually conceded to continuing fiber, probiotic, and avoiding dietary triggers, though she resented it.

She thought I was restricting her diet, when I was actually only adjusting it to avoid foods she couldn't tolerate. I found it interesting that even in the presence of colon cancer, she was still resistant to taking fiber and probiotics, as well as making other minor dietary changes.

She actually told me, "You should talk to my doctor about your treatments because he is not supporting my use of probiotics and fiber." Unfortunately, this sort of belief system is what I commonly see amongst healthcare professionals. Even though the microbiome protocols work well for someone, and resolve many of their health problems, healthcare professionals don't buy in, and therefore their patients don't buy in. They still want to go back to their previous habits and believe that they won't need to maintain their microbiome at all. That's why altering someone's mindset and habits are key to lifelong health.

This is also why we're in a mess with our current healthcare system. The mindset is, "I just need to take one more pill to solve all of my problems," instead of focusing on changing and improving behaviors long-term.

Microbiome changes are long-term improvements and don't happen as rapidly as someone might see by taking a prescribed narcotic, for example. People with this frame of thinking believe that the gut is something that can be "cured," and once that happens, they can do what they wish, like eating junk food, without repercussions.

However, the microbiome requires consistent maintenance to stay healthy. It's resilient to some junk food, but not a constant barrage of it. It must be maintained like any other organ in the body.

CASE #6 — MICROBIOME AND MIGRAINES

Review of Systems/Background:
- 31-year-old woman
- Very severe chronic migraines (severe nausea, vomiting)
- Chronic stress and anxiety
- Poor sleep
- Vitamin B12 deficiency
- Hypothyroidism
- Gas & bloating, some diarrhea (upon eating vegetables like garlic & onions especially)

Treating migraines can prove difficult, as it's dependent on many factors, such as diet, hormonal fluctuations, nutrient levels, and environmental triggers.

Allergies/Sensitivities:
No known allergies

Medical History:
- Migraines
- Hormonal Imbalances
- Intracranial Hypertension (previous pituitary tumor)
- Hypothyroidism

Medications & Supplements:
- Metoprolol 25mg once daily
- Desiccated thyroid 60mg once daily
- Clonazepam 0.25mg once daily
- Vitamin D3 1000IU once daily
- Magnesium threonate 200mg once daily

Treatment:

- Low FODMAP diet (MONASH University)
- Candibactin BR 2 tablets twice daily
- S. Boulardii 1-2 capsules daily
- Candida Stop 3 capsules daily
- Continue XOS Factor (XOS, an oligosaccharide fiber, + Factor 4 Fibre) and probiotics
- Inositol (Sensitol) 2 capsules twice daily
- Magnesium threonate 1 capsule three times daily
- EstroSmart 2-4 capsules daily
- Vitamin B12 oral (methylcobalamin) 1000mcg daily

Follow-up (30 days):

- Significant reduction in severity of migraines

Migraines were not resolved. She still had the same frequency, but the severity reduced from a pain scale of 8/10 to 5/10 with diet and magnesium threonate.

- Low FODMAP diet improved her gas & bloating

She noticed a difference with the microbiome shifts. In future, we could also try phosphatidylcholine to improve membrane stability for migraines. Remember that we need to ensure that she has a healthy microbiome before we give choline though, so as to prevent cardiotoxicity.

Summary:

This is another example of a gut-brain connection. However, in this case, it pertains to migraines. This case also showed the effectiveness of magnesium, in particular, magnesium threonate, in treating migraines and headaches. We love magnesium here at NutriChem!

CASE #7 — GENETIC CONDITIONS AND MICROBIOME

Review of Systems/Background:

- 43-year-old male
- Lives in group home for the mentally disabled
- Prader-Willi Syndrome (genetic condition), leading to numerous health problems
- Many psychological problems
- Many digestive problems, food allergies, and sensitivities
- Severe anxiety
- Obesity
- Learning Disabilities
- ADHD
- Adrenal insufficiency
- Chronic back pain

In the conventional healthcare system, you would deal with this patient by prescribing more drugs. An SSRI for anxiety, Imodium (loperamide) for diarrhea, Nexium (esomeprazole) for acid reflux, painkillers for chronic pain, anti-inflammatory drugs for inflammation and pain, allergy pills, CPAP machine for sleep apnea, benzodiazepines to help with sleep and anxiety, and so on.

By the time you got done, this guy would be so heavily medicated with drugs and devices that he wouldn't know what was happening in the real world, which is where he was in his life (he lived in a psychiatric group home for most of his life). When medications were used, he was essentially just sedated and sat quietly all day.

This group home was very resistant to dietary changes, primarily because they were difficult for the staff and roommates to implement. However, he responded extremely well to dietary changes. When he was younger, he lived with a vegetarian family and did very well, and he also responded really well to probiotics.

This man showed evidence that he functioned better on a healthy diet, but no one believed him, and instead, continued to pump him full of medications, lock him up in a mental institution, and feed him processed foods with minimal nutritional value. All this while bringing in more and more doctors and specialists to "fix" him with pharmaceuticals.

The barrier I see often in these sorts of cases is the illusion of higher cost to treat patients with a healthier diet plan. It "appears" to be a lot of work to change the diet, but what's the costs for those who stay in prisons, group homes, or institutions? Many drugs are also very expensive, and polypharmacy can cost patients and insurance companies many thousands of dollars a year. Over time, a healthy diet is by far the more cost-effective option for many of these institutionalized individuals. I often wonder how patients like this would fare in institutions that actually fed them microbiome-healthy foods.

Allergies/Sensitivities:
- Numerous severe food allergies
- Severe allergies to dairy & yeast

Medical History:
* Very Extensive!
- Prader-Willi Syndrome
- Severe Food Allergies
- Seasonal Allergies
- Addington's Disorder (Adrenal Insufficiency)
- Irritable Bowel Syndrome (IBS)
- Chronic Acid Reflux/GERD
- Anxiety Disorder
- Chronic Back & Knee Pain
- Obesity
- Many digestive issues (heartburn & gas)

Medications & Supplements

- Centrum Multi-vitamin once daily
- Cetirizine 20mg once daily
- Clonazepam 0.5mg once daily
- Cortef 30mg once daily
- Esomeprazole 40mg once daily
- Zinc citrate 50mg once daily
- Omega 3-6-9 x 2 capsules once daily
- Vitamin D3 1000IU once daily
- Megazyme Pro (Digestive Enzymes) 1 capsule once daily
- Acetaminophen 325mg as needed for pain
- Lorazepam 1mg as needed for anxiety
- Diphenhydramine 25mg as needed
- Beano 13.8mg as needed

Notice how many drugs this person is taking, and this is not even an exceptional case!

Treatment:

- Modified Paleo Diet (Gut Makeover Diet)
- Reduce and stop all diet soft drinks

Artificial sweeteners are bad for the microbiome despite no sugar calories.

- Re-introduce probiotics- NutriChem's *Nutridophilus* 1-2 caps twice daily
- Gradually reduce and discontinue esomeprazole, as bowel function improves
- Magnesium sulfate Gel (Mega Mag Gel) for back and knee pain—apply as needed
- Vitamin D 4000IU daily

Follow-up (30 days):

- Gut & overall health improved

Additional comments: He improved, but he was not able to continue his protocols and improvement of health because his group was not supportive. It was not sustainable to continue our protocols. This is a good example of a "failure" due to no support in place. Also, probiotics and fibers are not covered by the government healthcare plan, so he could not continue these supplements. Meanwhile, he continued using all of his drugs because they were covered by his healthcare plan. His inappropriate list of drugs was paid for, but the products that actually helped him were not covered and therefore not continued. This is the case with many of these institutionalized patients. Microbiome protocols are sometimes not sustainable because they are not covered by healthcare plans or insurance, and they require buy-in from surrounding social support or healthcare workers. There is a huge machine in place to give people drugs, but no system to help their microbiome, even if they wanted microbiome treatments desperately. This patient improved, but it was just not sustainable given the state of our current healthcare system.

Summary:
Just as in the past, when he would eat a vegetarian or paleo diet, his gut and overall health would improve.

REFERENCES

Adams LM, Turk DC. Psychosocial factors and central sensitivity syndromes. *Curr Rheumatol Rev*. 2015;11(2):96-108.

Agabio R.. Thiamine administration in alcohol dependent patients. *Alcohol and Alcoholism*. Volume 40, Issue 2, 1 March 2005, Pages 155–156, https://doi.org/10.1093/alcalc/agh106

Al-Saeed A. Gastrointestinal and Cardiovascular Risk of Nonsteroidal Anti-inflammatory Drugs. *Oman Med J*. 2011;26(6):385-91.

Amirian ES, Petrosino JF, Ajami NJ, Liu Y, Mims MP, Scheurer ME. Potential role of gastrointestinal microbiota composition in prostate cancer risk. *Infect Agent Cancer*. 2013;8(1):42. Published 2013 Nov 4. doi:10.1186/1750-9378-8-42

Anders HJ et al. The intestinal microbiota, a leaky gut, and abnormal immunity in kidney disease. *Kidney Int*. 2013 Jun;83(6):1010-6. doi: 10.1038/ki.2012.440. Epub 2013 Jan 16.

Arrieta MC, Bistritz L, Meddings JB. Alterations in intestinal permeability. *Gut*. 2006;55(10):1512-20.

Bailey MT, Coe CL. Endometriosis is associated with an altered profile of intestinal microflora in female rhesus monkeys. *Hum Reprod*. 2002 Jul;17(7):1704-8.

Baker, James M. et al. Estrogen–gut microbiome axis: Physiological and clinical implications. Maturitas 2017, Volume 103, 45 – 53.

Baker, L. et al. The role of estrogen in cardiovascular disease. *J Surg Res.* 2003 Dec;115(2):325-44. DOI: https://doi.org/10.1016/S0022-4804(03)00215-4

Biagi E, Candela M, Centanni M, et al. Gut microbiome in Down syndrome. *PLoS One.* 2014;9(11):e112023. Published 2014 Nov 11. doi:10.1371/journal.pone.0112023

Blaser M. Antibiotic overuse: stop the killing of beneficial bacteria. *Nature* volume 476, pages 393–394 (25 August 2011). https://www.nature.com/articles/476393a

Bonaz B, Bazin T, Pellissier S. The Vagus Nerve at the Interface of the Microbiota-Gut-Brain Axis. *Front Neurosci.* 2018; 12:49. Published 2018 Feb 7. doi:10.3389/fnins.2018.00049

Brandwein M, Steinberg D, Meshner S. Microbial biofilms and the human skin microbiome. *NPJ Biofilms Microbiomes.* 2016;2:3. Published 2016 Nov 23. doi:10.1038/s41522-016-0004-z

Breit S, Kupferberg A, Rogler G, Hasler G. Vagus Nerve as Modulator of the Brain-Gut Axis in Psychiatric and Inflammatory Disorders. *Front Psychiatry.* 2018;9:44. Published 2018 Mar 13. doi:10.3389/fpsyt.2018.00044

Buettner D, Skemp S. Blue Zones: Lessons From the World's Longest Lived. *Am J Lifestyle Med.* 2016;10(5):318-321. Published 2016 Jul 7. doi:10.1177/1559827616637066

Bull MJ, Plummer NT. Part 1: The Human Gut Microbiome in Health and Disease. *Integr Med (Encinitas).* 2014;13(6):17-22.

Bull MJ, Plummer NT. Part 2: Treatments for Chronic Gastrointestinal Disease and Gut Dysbiosis. *Integr Med (Encinitas).* 2015;14(1):25-33.

Butler MI, Cryan JF, Dinan TG. Man and the Microbiome: A New Theory of Everything? *Annual Review of Clinical Psychology.* 2019 15:1.

Calton JB. Prevalence of micronutrient deficiency in popular diet plans. *J Int Soc Sports Nutr.* 2010;7:24. Published 2010 Jun 10. doi:10.1186/1550-2783-7-24

Cámara-Lemarroy CR, Rodriguez-Gutierrez R, Monreal-Robles R, Marfil-Rivera A. Gastrointestinal disorders associated with migraine: A comprehensive review. *World J Gastroenterol.* 2016;22(36):8149-60.

Canadian Institute for Health 2017. *Alcohol Harm in Canada: Health Report 2017.* *https://www.cihi.ca/sites/default/files/document/report-alcohol-hospitalizations-en-web.pdf*

Canadian Institute for Health 2018. *Drug Spending at a Glance 2018 Health Report.* https://www.cihi.ca/sites/default/files/document/nhex-drug-infosheet-2018-en-web.pdf

Cani PD et al. Endocannabinoids — at the crossroads between the gut microbiota and host metabolism. *Nature Reviews Endocrinology* volume 12, pages 133–143 (2016)

Carabotti M, Scirocco A, Maselli MA, Severi C. The gut-brain axis: interactions between enteric microbiota, central and enteric nervous systems. *Ann Gastroenterol.* 2015;28(2):203-209.

Cartwright C, Gibson K, Read J, Cowan O, Dehar T. Long-term antidepressant use: patient perspectives of benefits and adverse effects. *Patient Prefer Adherence.* 2016;10:1401-7. Published 2016 Jul 28. doi:10.2147/PPA.S110632

Carlson JL, Erickson JM, Lloyd BB, Slavin JL. Health Effects and Sources of Prebiotic Dietary Fiber. *Curr Dev Nutr.* 2018;2(3):nzy005. Published 2018 Jan 29. doi:10.1093/cdn/nzy005

Chandra H, Bishnoi P, Yadav A, Patni B, Mishra AP, Nautiyal AR. Antimicrobial Resistance and the Alternative Resources with Special Emphasis on Plant-Based Antimicrobials-A Review. *Plants (Basel).* 2017;6(2):16. Published 2017 Apr 10. doi:10.3390/plants6020016

Choung RS, Locke GR, Zinsmeister AR, Schleck CD, Talley NJ. Psychosocial distress and somatic symptoms in community subjects with irritable bowel syndrome: a psychological component is the rule. *Am J Gastroenterol.* 2009;104(7):1772-9.

Chu M, Zhang MB, Liu YC, et al. Role of Berberine in the Treatment of Methicillin-Resistant Staphylococcus aureus Infections. *Sci Rep.* 2016;6:24748. Published 2016 Apr 22. doi:10.1038/srep24748

Clarke G, Stilling RM, Kennedy PJ, Stanton C, Cryan JF, Dinan TG. Minireview: Gut microbiota: the neglected endocrine organ. *Mol Endocrinol.* 2014;28(8):1221-38.

Clapp M, Aurora N, Herrera L, Bhatia M, Wilen E, Wakefield S. Gut microbiota's effect on mental health: The gut-brain axis. *Clin Pract.* 2017;7(4):987. Published 2017 Sep 15. doi:10.4081/cp.2017.987

Cluny NL. Cannabinoid signalling regulates inflammation and energy balance: The importance of the brain–gut axis. *Brain, Behavior, and Immunity*; July 2012; 26 (5); pg. 691-698.

Cook CCH et al. B Vitamin Deficiency and Neuropsychiatric Syndromes in Alcohol Misuse. *Alcohol and Alcoholism*, Volume 33, Issue 4, 1 July 1998, Pages 317- 336. https://doi.org/10.1093/oxfordjournals.alcalc.a008400

Cryan JF. Stress and the Microbiota-Gut-Brain Axis: An Evolving Concept in Psychiatry. *Can J Psychiatry.* 2016;61(4):201-3.

Depot-medroxyprogesterone acetate (DMPA) and cancer: memorandum from a WHO meeting. *Bull World Health Organ.* 1993;71(6):669-76.

Dulantha U et al. Regulation of Tight Junction Permeability by Intestinal Bacteria and Dietary Components, *The Journal of Nutrition*, Volume 141, Issue 5, 1 May 2011, Pages 769–776, https://doi.org/10.3945/jn.110.135657

Eisenstein M. Nutrition Digest: Digestive Issues. *American Nutrition Association.* Article from *NOHA NEWS*, Summer 2007. Volume 38 No.2. http://americannutritionassociation.org/newsletter/digestive-issues

Ellermann M, Sartor RB. Intestinal bacterial biofilms modulate mucosal immune responses. *J Immunol Sci.* 2018;2(2):13-18.

Farzi A, Fröhlich EE, Holzer P. Gut Microbiota and the Neuroendocrine System. *Neurotherapeutics.* 2018;15(1):5-22.

Ferguson JM. SSRI Antidepressant Medications: Adverse Effects and Tolerability. *Prim Care Companion J Clin Psychiatry.* 2001;3(1):22-27.

Frassetto LA et al. Metabolic and physiologic improvements from consuming a paleolithic, hunter-gatherer type diet. Eur J Clin Nutr. 2009 Aug;63(8):947-55. doi: 10.1038/ejcn.2009.4. Epub 2009 Feb 11.

Francino MP. Antibiotics and the Human Gut Microbiome: Dysbioses and Accumulation of Resistances. *Front Microbiol.* 2016;6:1543. Published 2016 Jan 12. doi:10.3389/fmicb.2015.01543

Foster JA, Rinaman L, Cryan JF. Stress & the gut-brain axis: Regulation by the microbiome. *Neurobiol Stress.* 2017;7:124-136. Published 2017 Mar 19. doi:10.1016/j.ynstr.2017.03.001

Fuhrman B. et al. Associations of the Fecal Microbiome With Urinary Estrogens and Estrogen Metabolites in Postmenopausal Women, *The Journal of Clinical Endocrinology & Metabolism*, Volume 99, Issue 12, 1 December 2014, Pages 4632–4640, https://doi.org/10.1210/jc.2014-2222

Galland L. The gut microbiome and the brain. *J Med Food.* 2014;17(12):1261-72.

Gibson MK, Crofts TS, Dantas G. Antibiotics and the developing infant gut microbiota and resistome. *Curr Opin Microbiol.* 2015;27:51-6.

Gilbert JA, et al. Current understanding of the human microbiome. *Nature Medicine* **volume 24**, pages 392–400 (2018). doi: 10.1038/nm.4517.

Giloteaux L et al. Reduced diversity and altered composition of the gut microbiome in individuals with myalgic encephalomyelitis/chronic fatigue syndrome. *Microbiome* 2016 4:30. https://doi.org/10.1186/s40168-016-0171-4

Gomez-Arango LF, et al. Connections Between the Gut Microbiome and Metabolic Hormones in Early Pregnancy in Overweight and Obese Women. Diabetes Aug 2016, 65 (8) 2214-2223; DOI: 10.2337/db16-0278

Griffin JL, Wang X, Stanley E. Does our gut microbiome predict cardio-vascular risk? A review of the evidence from metabolomics. *Circ Cardiovasc Genet.* 2015;8(1):187-91.

Guo Y, Qi Y, Yang X, Zhao L, Wen S, Liu Y, et al. (2016) Association between Polycystic Ovary Syndrome and Gut Microbiota. *PLoS ONE* 11(4): e0153196. https://doi.org/10.1371/journal.pone.0153196

Haastrup PF, et al. Side Effects of Long-Term Proton Pump Inhibitor Use: A Review. *Basic Clin Pharmacol Toxicol.* 2018 Aug;123(2):114-121. doi: 10.1111/bcpt.13023. Epub 2018 May 24.

Hadar Neuman, Justine W. Debelius, Rob Knight, Omry Koren; Microbial endocrinology: the interplay between the microbiota and the endocrine system, *FEMS Microbiology Reviews*, Volume 39, Issue 4, 1 July 2015, Pages 509–521, https://doi.org/10.1093/femsre/fuu010

Harada N, Hanaoka R, Hanada K, Izawa T, Inui H, Yamaji R. Hypogonadism alters cecal and fecal microbiota in male mice. *Gut Microbes.* 2016;7(6):533-539.

Haro C, Rangel-Zúñiga OA, Alcalá-Díaz JF, et al. Intestinal Microbiota Is Influenced by Gender and Body Mass Index. *PLoS One.* 2016;11(5):e0154090. Published 2016 May 26. doi:10.1371/journal.pone.0154090

Hays MT. Thyroid hormone and the gut. *Endocr Res.* 1988;14(2-3):203-24.

Hibberd MC, Wu M, Rodionov DA, et al. The effects of micronutrient deficiencies on bacterial species from the human gut microbiota. *Sci Transl Med.* 2017;9(390):eaal4069.

Hill JM, Bhattacharjee S, Pogue AI, Lukiw WJ. The gastrointestinal tract microbiome and potential link to Alzheimer's disease. *Front Neurol.* 2014;5:43. Published 2014 Apr 4. doi:10.3389/fneur.2014.00043

Ho, Pochu et al. More Than a Gut Feeling: The Implications of the Gut Microbiota in Psychiatry. *Biological Psychiatry*, Volume 81, Issue 5, e35 - e37

Hollander D. Intestinal permeability, leaky gut, and intestinal disorders. Curr Gastroenterol Rep. 1999 Oct;1(5):410-6.

Holscher HD. Dietary fiber and prebiotics and the gastrointestinal microbiota. *Gut Microbes.* 2017;8(2):172-184.

Holzer P, Farzi A. Neuropeptides and the microbiota-gut-brain axis. *Adv Exp Med Biol.* 2014;817:195-219.

Hoyne GF. Microbial dysbiosis and disease pathogenesis of endometriosis, could there be a link?. Allied J Med Res 2017;1(1):1-9.

Hoyumpa AM. Mechanisms of vitamin deficiencies in alcoholism. *Alcohol Clin Exp Res.* 1986 Dec;10(6):573-81.

Hsieh MH, Versalovic J. The human microbiome and probiotics: implications for pediatrics. *Curr Probl Pediatr Adolesc Health Care.* 2008;38(10):309-27.

Iadecola C. Sugar and Alzheimer's disease: a bittersweet truth. *Nat Neurosci.* 2015;18(4):477-8.

Indrio F, Neu J. The intestinal microbiome of infants and the use of probiotics. *Curr Opin Pediatr.* 2011;23(2):145-50.

International Foundation for Gastrointestinal Disorders. *Facts about Irritable Bowel Syndrome (IBS).* Last updated Nov 24, 2016. https://www.aboutibs.org/facts-about-ibs.html

Jandhyala SM, Talukdar R, Subramanyam C, Vuyyuru H, Sasikala M, Nageshwar Reddy D. Role of the normal gut microbiota. *World J Gastroenterol.* 2015;21(29):8787-803.

Javurek AB, Spollen WG, Johnson SA, et al. Effects of exposure to bisphenol A and ethinyl estradiol on the gut microbiota of parents and their offspring in a rodent model. *Gut Microbes.* 2016;7(6):471-485.

Jernberg C et al. Long-term impacts of antibiotic exposure on the human intestinal microbiota. Microbiology. 2010 Nov;156(Pt 11):3216-23. doi: 10.1099/mic.0.040618-0. Epub 2010 Aug 12.

Jia JP et al. Differential acetylcholine and choline concentrations in the cerebrospinal fluid of patients with Alzheimer's disease and vascular dementia. Chin Med J (Engl). 2004 Aug;117(8):1161-4.

Jones MR, Viswanath O, Peck J, Kaye AD, Gill JS, Simopoulos TT. A Brief History of the Opioid Epidemic and Strategies for Pain Medicine. *Pain Ther.* 2018;7(1):13-21.

Karl JP, Hatch AM, Arcidiacono SM, et al. Effects of Psychological, Environmental and Physical Stressors on the Gut Microbiota. *Front Microbiol.* 2018;9:2013. Published 2018 Sep 11. doi:10.3389/fmicb.2018.02013

Kau AL, Ahern PP, Griffin NW, Goodman AL, Gordon JI. Human nutrition, the gut microbiome and the immune system. *Nature.* 2011;474(7351):327-36. Published 2011 Jun 15. doi:10.1038/nature10213

Khanna, Sahil; Tosh, Pritish K. A Clinician's Primer on the Role of the Microbiome in Human Health and Disease. *Mayo Clinic Proceedings.* 2014;89(1):107-114.

Kho ZY, Lal SK. The Human Gut Microbiome - A Potential Controller of Wellness and Disease. *Front Microbiol.* 2018; 9:1835. Published 2018 Aug 14. doi:10.3389/fmicb.2018.01835

Kirsten Tillisch (2014) The effects of gut microbiota on CNS function in humans, Gut Microbes, 5:3,404-410, DOI: 10.4161/gmic.29232

Kuntz TM and Gilbert JA. Introducing the Microbiome into Precision Medicine. *Trends Pharmacol Sci.* 2017 Jan;38(1):81-91. doi: 10.1016/j.tips.2016.10.001. Epub 2016 Nov 1.

Kwa M, Plottel CS, Blaser MJ, Adams S. The Intestinal Microbiome and Estrogen Receptor-Positive Female Breast Cancer. *J Natl Cancer Inst.* 2016;108(8):djw029. Published 2016 Apr 22. doi:10.1093/jnci/djw029

Lach, G., Schellekens, H., Dinan, T.G. et al. Anxiety, Depression, and the Microbiome: A Role for Gut Peptides. *Neurotherapeutics* (2018) 15: 36. https://doi.org/10.1007/s13311-017-0585-0

Langdon A, Crook N, Dantas G. The effects of antibiotics on the microbiome throughout development and alternative approaches for therapeutic modulation. *Genome Med.* 2016;8(1):39. Published 2016 Apr 13. doi:10.1186/s13073-016-0294-z

Lawrence K, Hyde J. Microbiome restoration diet improves digestion, cognition and physical and emotional wellbeing. *PLoS One.* 2017;12(6):e0179017. Published 2017 Jun 14. doi:10.1371/journal.pone.0179017

Leclercq S et al. Intestinal permeability, gut-bacterial dysbiosis, and behavioral markers of alcohol-dependence severity. *PNAS* October 21, 2014 111 (42) E4485-E4493; published ahead of print October 6, 2014 https://doi.org/10.1073/pnas.1415174111

Lee, S. et al. Irritable Bowel Syndrome is strongly associated with generalized anxiety disorder: a community study. 2009 Sep 15;30(6):643-51. doi: 10.1111/j.1365-2036.2009.04074.x. Epub 2009 Jun 23

Lerner A, Jeremias P, Matthias T. Gut-thyroid axis and celiac disease. *Endocr Connect.* 2017;6(4):R52-R58.

Lerner A, Neidhöfer S, Matthias T. The Gut Microbiome Feelings of the Brain: A Perspective for Non-Microbiologists. *Microorganisms.* 2017;5(4):66. Published 2017 Oct 12. doi:10.3390/microorganisms5040066

Ley R, et al. Microbial ecology: human gut microbes associated with obesity. *Nature* volume 444, pages 1022–1023 (21 December 2006)

Li CI, Beaber EF, Tang MT, Porter PL, Daling JR, Malone KE. Effect of depo-medroxyprogesterone acetate on breast cancer risk among women 20 to 44 years of age. *Cancer Res.* 2012;72(8):2028-35.

Li, Jau-Yi et al. Sex steroid deficiency-associated bone loss is microbiota dependent and prevented by probiotics. *Clin Invest.* 2016;126(6):2049-2063. https://doi.org/10.1172/JCI86062.

Liang D, Leung RK, Guan W, Au WW. Involvement of gut microbiome in human health and disease: brief overview, knowledge gaps and research opportunities. *Gut Pathog.* 2018;10:3. Published 2018 Jan 25. doi:10.1186/s13099-018-0230-4

Lievertz RW. Pharmacology and pharmacokinetics of estrogens. *American Journal of Obstetrics and Gynecology.* Volume 156, Issue 5, May 1987, Pages 1289-1293

Lindheim L, Bashir M, Münzker J, Trummer C, Zachhuber V, Leber B, et al. (2017) Alterations in Gut Microbiome Composition and Barrier Function Are Associated with Reproductive and Metabolic Defects in Women with Polycystic Ovary Syndrome (PCOS): A Pilot Study. *PLoS ONE* 12(1): e0168390. https://doi.org/10.1371/journal.pone.0168390

Lizcano F, Guzmán G. Estrogen Deficiency and the Origin of Obesity during Menopause. *Biomed Res Int.* 2014;2014:757461.

Lloyd-Price J, Abu-Ali G, Huttenhower C. The healthy human microbiome. *Genome Med.* 2016;8(1):51. Published 2016 Apr 27. doi:10.1186/s13073-016-0307-y

Lubin FD, Campbell SL. A Gut Feeling About Seizures. *Epilepsy Curr.* 2018;18(6):389-390.

Lucas SM et al. The role of inflammation in CNS injury and disease. *British Journal of Pharmacology* (2006) 147, S232–S240. doi:10.1038/sj.bjp.0706400

Luchsinger JA, Gustafson DR. Adiposity, type 2 diabetes, and Alzheimer's disease. *J Alzheimers Dis.* 2009;16(4):693-704.

Mach N, Clark A. Micronutrient Deficiencies and the Human Gut Microbiota. *Trends in Microbiology.* Volume 25, Issue 8; pg. 607-610. Published August 2017. https://doi.org/10.1016/j.tim.2017.06.004

Magnúsdóttir S, Ravcheev D, de Crécy-Lagard V, Thiele I. Systematic genome assessment of B-vitamin biosynthesis suggests co-operation among gut microbes. *Front Genet.* 2015;6:148. Published 2015 Apr 20. doi:10.3389/fgene.2015.00148

Manson JE, Chlebowski RT, Stefanick ML, et al. Menopausal hormone therapy and health outcomes during the intervention and extended poststopping phases of the Women's Health Initiative randomized trials. *JAMA*. 2013;310(13):1353-68.

Manzardo AM, He J, Poje A, Penick EC, Campbell J, Butler MG. Double-blind, randomized placebo-controlled clinical trial of benfotiamine for severe alcohol dependence. *Drug Alcohol Depend*. 2013;133(2):562-70.

Manzardo AM, Pendleton T, Poje A, Penick EC, Butler MG. Change in psychiatric symptomatology after benfotiamine treatment in males is related to lifetime alcoholism severity. *Drug Alcohol Depend*. 2015;152:257-63.

Manzoor MAP, Rekha PD. Prostate cancer: Microbiome- the "unforeseen organ." Nat Rev Urol. 2017 Sep;14(9):521-522. doi: 10.1038/nrurol.2017.97. Epub 2017 Jun 27.

Marchesi JR, Adams DH, Fava F, et al. The gut microbiota and host health: a new clinical frontier. *Gut*. 2015;65(2):330-9.

Markowiak P, Śliżewska K. Effects of Probiotics, Prebiotics, and Synbiotics on Human Health. *Nutrients*. 2017;9(9):1021. Published 2017 Sep 15. doi:10.3390/nu9091021

Mariotti A. The effects of chronic stress on health: new insights into the molecular mechanisms of brain-body communication. *Future Sci OA*. 2015;1(3):FSO23. Published 2015 Nov 1. doi:10.4155/fso.15.21

Matsui H, Shimokawa O, Kaneko T, Nagano Y, Rai K, Hyodo I. The pathophysiology of non-steroidal anti-inflammatory drug (NSAID)-induced mucosal injuries in stomach and small intestine. *J Clin Biochem Nutr*. 2011;48(2):107-11.

Mehrpouya-Bahrami P. Blockade of CB1 cannabinoid receptor alters gut microbiota and attenuates inflammation and diet-induced obesity. *Scientific Reports* volume 7, Article number: 15645 (2017)

Mendelsohn AR and Larrick JW. Dietary modification of the microbiome affects risk for cardiovascular disease. Rejuvenation Res. 2013 Jun;16(3):241-4. doi: 10.1089/rej.2013.1447.

Mishra BN. Secret of eternal youth; teaching from the centenarian hot spots ("blue zones"). *Indian J Community Med*. 2009;34(4):273-5.

Morrison DJ, Preston T. Formation of short chain fatty acids by the gut microbiota and their impact on human metabolism. *Gut Microbes.* 2016;7(3):189-200.

Mu Q, Kirby J, Reilly CM, Luo XM. Leaky Gut as a Danger Signal for Autoimmune Diseases. *Front Immunol.* 2017;8:598. Published 2017 May 23. doi:10.3389/fimmu.2017.00598

Mueller NT, Bakacs E, Combellick J, Grigoryan Z, Dominguez-Bello MG. The infant microbiome development: mom matters. *Trends Mol Med.* 2014;21(2):109-17.

Murtaza N et al. Diet and the Microbiome. *Gastroenterol Clin North Am.* 2017 Mar;46(1):49-60. doi: 10.1016/j.gtc.2016.09.005. Epub 2017 Jan 4.

National Institute on Alcohol Abuse and Alcoholism. *Alcohol Facts & Statistics.* Updated 2018.

https://www.niaaa.nih.gov/alcohol-health/overview-alcohol-consumption/alcohol-facts-and-statistics

Nehra AK, et al. Proton Pump Inhibitors: Review of Emerging Concerns. *Mayo Clin Proc.* 2018 Feb;93(2):240-246. doi: 10.1016/j.mayocp.2017.10.022.

Nelles JL, Hu WY, Prins GS. Estrogen action and prostate cancer. *Expert Rev Endocrinol Metab.* 2011;6(3):437-451.

O'Mahony SM et al. Serotonin, tryptophan metabolism and the brain-gut-microbiome axis. Behavioural Brain Research. 2015; 277; 32-48.

Paganini D, Uyoga MA, Zimmermann MB. Iron Fortification of Foods for Infants and Children in Low-Income Countries: Effects on the Gut Microbiome, Gut Inflammation, and Diarrhea. *Nutrients.* 2016;8(8):494. Published 2016 Aug 12. doi:10.3390/nu8080494

Pandey KR, Naik SR, Vakil BV. Probiotics, prebiotics and synbiotics- a review. *J Food Sci Technol.* 2015;52(12):7577-87.

Paul C, Skegg DC, Spears GF. Depot medroxyprogesterone (Depo-Provera) and risk of breast cancer. *BMJ.* 1989;299(6702):759-62.

Poutahidis T, Springer A, Levkovich T, et al. Probiotic microbes sustain youthful serum testosterone levels and testicular size in aging mice. *PLoS One.* 2014;9(1):e84877. Published 2014 Jan 2. doi:10.1371/journal.pone.0084877

Powers MS et al. Pharmacokinetics and pharmacodynamics of transdermal dosage forms of 17 beta-estradiol: comparison with conventional oral estrogens used for hormone replacement. *Am J Obstet Gynecol.* 1985 Aug 15;152(8):1099-106.

Preidis GA, Versalovic J. Targeting the human microbiome with antibiotics, probiotics, and prebiotics: gastroenterology enters the metagenomics era. *Gastroenterology.* 2009;136(6):2015-31.

Rahmoune H, Boutrid N. Migraine, Celiac Disease and Intestinal Microbiota. *Pediatr Neurol Briefs.* 2017;31(2):6.

Rajendran P, et al. The multifaceted link between inflammation and human diseases. J Cell Physiol. 2018 Sep;233(9):6458-6471. doi: 10.1002/jcp.26479. Epub 2018 Mar 7.

Rea K, Dinan TG, Cryan JF. The microbiome: A key regulator of stress and neuroinflammation. *Neurobiol Stress.* 2016;4:23-33. Published 2016 Mar 4. doi:10.1016/j.ynstr.2016.03.001

Rezac S, Kok CR, Heermann M, Hutkins R. Fermented Foods as a Dietary Source of Live Organisms. *Front Microbiol.* 2018;9:1785. Published 2018 Aug 24. doi:10.3389/fmicb.2018.01785

Rietjens IMCM, Louisse J, Beekmann K. The potential health effects of dietary phytoestrogens. *Br J Pharmacol.* 2016;174(11):1263-1280.

Rowland I, Gibson G, Heinken A, et al. Gut microbiota functions: metabolism of nutrients and other food components. *Eur J Nutr.* 2017;57(1):1-24.

Rummans TA et al. How Good Intentions Contributed to Bad Outcomes: The Opioid Crisis. *Mayo Clinic Proceedings.* March 2018 Volume 93, Issue 3, Pages 344–350.

Russell RI. Non-steroidal anti-inflammatory drugs and gastrointestinal damage-problems and solutions. *Postgrad Med J.* 2001;77(904):82-8.

Santarsieri D, Schwartz TL. Antidepressant efficacy and side-effect burden: a quick guide for clinicians. *Drugs Context*. 2015;4:212290. Published 2015 Oct 8. doi:10.7573/dic.212290

Serino M, Blasco-Baque V, Nicolas S, Burcelin R. Far from the eyes, close to the heart: dysbiosis of gut microbiota and cardiovascular consequences. *Curr Cardiol Rep*. 2014;16(11):540.

Shin H et al. The first microbial environment of infants born by C-section: the operating room microbes. *Microbiome* 2015; **3**:59. https://doi.org/10.1186/s40168-015-0126-1

Singh RK, Chang HW, Yan D, et al. Influence of diet on the gut microbiome and implications for human health. *J Transl Med*. 2017;15(1):73. Published 2017 Apr 8. doi:10.1186/s12967-017-1175-y

Singhal M, Turturice BA, Manzella CR, et al. Serotonin Transporter Deficiency is Associated with Dysbiosis and Changes in Metabolic Function of the Mouse Intestinal Microbiome. *Sci Rep*. 2019;9(1):2138. Published 2019 Feb 14. doi:10.1038/s41598-019-38489-8

Skonieczna-Żydecka K, Marlicz W, Misera A, Koulaouzidis A, Łoniewski I. Microbiome-The Missing Link in the Gut-Brain Axis: Focus on Its Role in Gastrointestinal and Mental Health. *J Clin Med*. 2018;7(12):521. Published 2018 Dec 7. doi:10.3390/jcm7120521

Skrypnik K, Suliburska J. Association between the gut microbiota and mineral metabolism. *J Sci Food Agric*. 2018 May; 98 (7): 2449-2460. 10.1002/jsfa.8724 Epub 2017 Oct 31.

Song MK, Bischoff DS, Song AM, Uyemura K, Yamaguchi DT. Metabolic relationship between diabetes and Alzheimer's Disease affected by Cyclo(His-Pro) plus zinc treatment. *BBA Clin*. 2016;7:41-54. Published 2016 Oct 2. doi:10.1016/j.bbacli.2016.09.003

Spencer MD, Hamp TJ, Reid RW, Fischer LM, Zeisel SH, Fodor AA. Association between composition of the human gastrointestinal microbiome and development of fatty liver with choline deficiency. *Gastroenterology*. 2010;140(3):976-86.

Spinelli E, Blackford R. Gut Microbiota, the Ketogenic Diet and Epilepsy. *Pediatr Neurol Briefs*. 2018;32:10. Published 2018 Sep 21. doi:10.15844/pedneurbriefs-32-10

Subramani R, Narayanasamy M, Feussner KD. Plant-derived antimicrobials to fight against multi-drug-resistant human pathogens. *3 Biotech*. 2017;7(3):172.

Sudo N. (2014) Microbiome, HPA Axis and Production of Endocrine Hormones in the Gut. In: Lyte M., Cryan J. (eds) Microbial Endocrinology: The Microbiota-Gut-Brain Axis in Health and Disease. Advances in Experimental Medicine and Biology, vol 817. Springer, New York, NY

Sweeney TE, Morton JM. The human gut microbiome: a review of the effect of obesity and surgically induced weight loss. *JAMA Surg*. 2013;148(6):563-9.

Tamburini S et al. The microbiome in early life: implications for health outcomes. *Nature Medicine* volume 22, pages 713–722 (2016)

Tang WH, Kitai T, Hazen SL. Gut Microbiota in Cardiovascular Health and Disease. *Circ Res*. 2017;120(7):1183-1196.

Tang M, Frank DN, Hendricks AE, et al. Iron in Micronutrient Powder Promotes an Unfavorable Gut Microbiota in Kenyan Infants. *Nutrients*. 2017;9(7):776. Published 2017 Jul 19. doi:10.3390/nu9070776

Thursby E, Juge N. Introduction to the human gut microbiota. *Biochem J*. 2017;474(11):1823-1836. Published 2017 May 16. doi:10.1042/BCJ20160510

Tremellen K, McPhee N, Pearce K, Benson S, Schedlowski M, Engler H. Role of Gut Microbiota and Gut-Brain and Gut-Liver Axes in Physiological Regulation of Inflammation, Energy Balance, and Metabolism. *Am J Physiol Endocrinol Metab*. 2017;314(3):E206-E213.

Tremlett H et al. The gut microbiome in human neurological disease: A review. Ann Neurol. 2017 Mar;81(3):369-382. doi: 10.1002/ana.24901. Epub 2017 Mar 20.

Urbaniak C, Gloor GB, Brackstone M, Scott L, Tangney M, Reid G. The Microbiota of Breast Tissue and Its Association with Breast Cancer. *Appl Environ Microbiol*. 2016;82(16):5039-48. Published 2016 Jul 29. doi:10.1128/AEM.01235-16

Vaezi MF et al. Complications of Proton Pump Inhibitor Therapy. *Gastroenterology*. 2017 Jul;153(1):35-48. doi: 10.1053/j.gastro.2017.04.047. Epub 2017 May 19.

van Hemert S, Breedveld AC, Rovers JM, et al. Migraine associated with gastrointestinal disorders: review of the literature and clinical implications. *Front Neurol.* 2014;5:241. Published 2014 Nov 21. doi:10.3389/fneur.2014.00241

Vahedi H, Ansari R, Mir-Nasseri M, Jafari E. Irritable bowel syndrome: a review article. *Middle East J Dig Dis.* 2010;2(2):66-77.

Velicer CM, Heckbert SR, Lampe JW, Potter JD, Robertson CA, Taplin SH. Antibiotic Use in Relation to the Risk of Breast Cancer. *JAMA.* 2004;291(7):827–835. doi:10.1001/jama.291.7.827

Vieira AT, Castelo PM, Ribeiro DA, Ferreira CM. Influence of Oral and Gut Microbiota in the Health of Menopausal Women. *Front Microbiol.* 2017;8:1884. Published 2017 Sep 28. doi:10.3389/fmicb.2017.01884

Villa C, Ward W, and Comelli E (2017). Gut microbio-ta-bone axis, Critical Reviews in Food Science and Nutrition, 57:8, 1664-1672, DOI: 10.1080/10408398.2015.1010034

Virili C and Centanni M. Does microbiota composition affect thyroid homeostasis? *Endocrine.* 2015 Aug;49(3):583-7. doi: 10.1007/s12020-014-0509-2. Epub 2014 Dec 17.

Volvert ML, Seyen S, Piette M, et al. Benfotiamine, a synthetic S-acyl thiamine derivative, has different mechanisms of action and a different pharmacological profile than lipid-soluble thiamine disulfide derivatives. *BMC Pharmacol.* 2008;8:10. Published 2008 Jun 12. doi:10.1186/1471-2210-8-10

Walsh CJ, Guinane CM, O'Toole PW, Cotter PD. Beneficial modulation of the gut microbiota. *FEBS Letters.* 2014; 588 (22): 4120-4130.

Wang Y, Kasper LH. The role of microbiome in central nervous system disorders. *Brain Behav Immun.* 2013;38:1-12.

Ward E. Addressing nutritional gaps with multivitamin and mineral supplements. *Nutr J.* 2014;13:72. Published 2014 Jul 15. doi:10.1186/1475-2891-13-72

Weaver CM. Diet, gut microbiome, and bone health. *Curr Osteoporos Rep.* 2015;13(2):125-30.

Woolf CJ. Central sensitization: implications for the diagnosis and treatment of pain. *Pain.* 2010;152(3 Suppl): S2-15.

WHO- World Heath Organization. *News Release Special Report: Investing in treatment for depression and anxiety leads to fourfold return.* April 2016. https://www.who.int/news-room/detail/13-04-2016-investing-in-treatment-for-depression-and-anxiety-leads-to-fourfold-return

Wischmeyer PE, McDonald D, Knight R. Role of the microbiome, probiotics, and 'dysbiosis therapy' in critical illness. *Curr Opin Crit Care.* 2016;22(4):347-53.

Wright AT. Gut commensals make choline too. *Nat Microbiol.* 2019 Jan;4(1):4-5. doi: 10.1038/s41564-018-0325-1.

Xu X, Chen F, Huang Z, et al. Meeting report: a close look at oral biofilms and microbiomes. *Int J Oral Sci.* 2018;10(3):28. Published 2018 Aug 15. doi:10.1038/s41368-018-0030-1

Ya-Shu Kuang, et al. Connections between the human gut microbiome and gestational diabetes mellitus. *GigaScience*, Volume 6, Issue 8, 1 August 2017, gix058, https://doi.org/10.1093/gigascience/gix058

Yassour M, Vatanen T, Siljander H, et al. Natural history of the infant gut microbiome and impact of antibiotic treatment on bacterial strain diversity and stability. *Sci Transl Med.* 2016;8(343):343ra81.

Zhang J et al. Dysbiosis of the gut microbiome is associated with thyroid cancer and thyroid nodules and correlated with clinical index of thyroid function. Endocrine. 2018 Dec 24. doi: 10.1007/s12020-018-1831-x. [Epub ahead of print]

Zhao F et al. Alterations of the Gut Microbiota in Hashimoto's Thyroiditis Patients. *Thyroid.* 2018 Feb;28(2):175-186. doi: 10.1089/thy.2017.0395. Epub 2018 Feb 1.

Zhao J et al. Modeling the Impact of Antibiotic Exposure on Human Microbiota. *Scientific Reports* volume 4, Article number: 4345 (2014)

Zhu W, Wang Z, Tang WHW, Hazen SL. Gut Microbe-Generated Trimethylamine *N*-Oxide From Dietary Choline Is Prothrombotic in Subjects. *Circulation.* 2017;135(17):1671-1673.

NutriChem™
Personalized Health Solutions

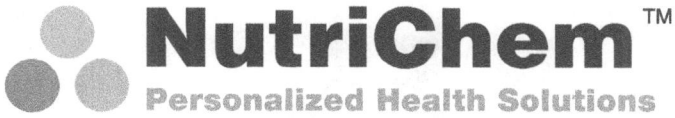

NUTRICHEM RECOMMENDED PRODUCTS

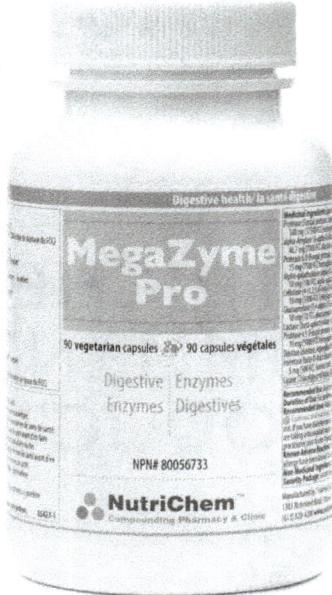

Bloated? Gassy? Indigestion after a big meal? Power up your digestion with MegaZyme Pro!

Purchase this product at www.nutrichem.com

NutriChem™
Personalized Health Solutions

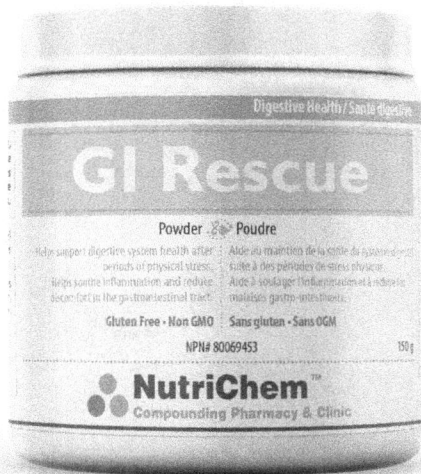

If you suffer from heartburn, reach
for something safer than antacids!

Purchase this product at www.nutrichem.com

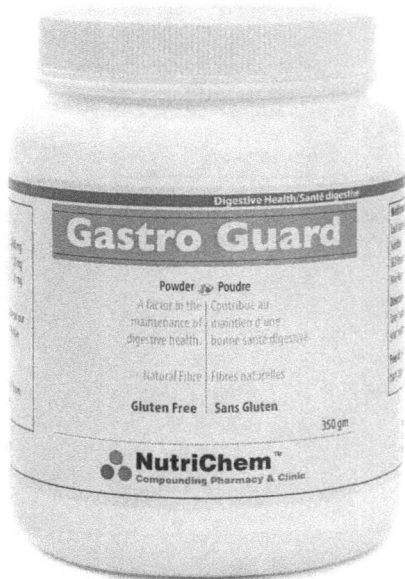

Soothe and fuel your
gut's microecosystem
with Gastro Guard!

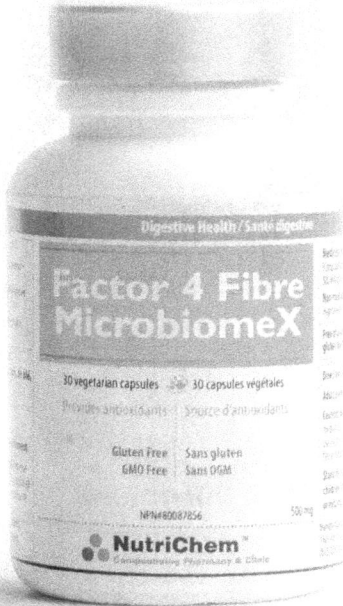

Feed your body's
healthy bacteria exactly
what they need!

Purchase this product at www.nutrichem.com

NutriChem™
Personalized Health Solutions

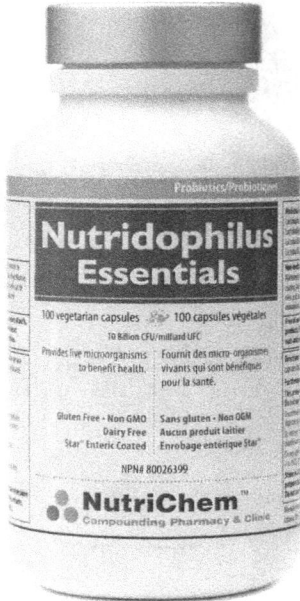

Upset stomach? Diarrhea? Soothe
your gut with Nutridophilus
Essentials probiotic

Purchase this product at www.nutrichem.com

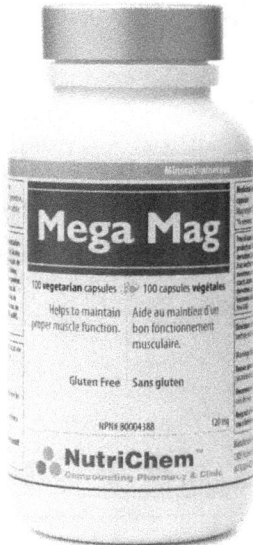

Magnesium is involved in over 300 essential biochemical processes in the human body. Most of us are not getting enough from our diet. Are you?

Purchase this product at www.nutrichem.com

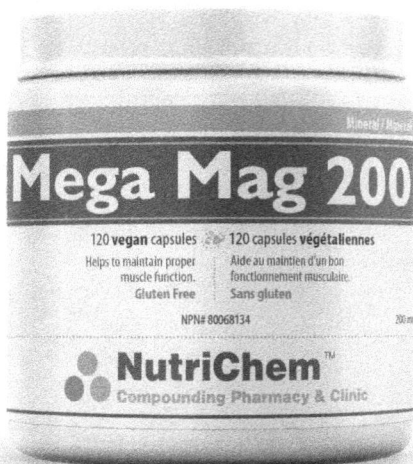

Magnesium is involved in over 300 essential biochemical processes in the human body. Most of us are not getting enough from our diet. Are you?

Purchase this product at www.nutrichem.com

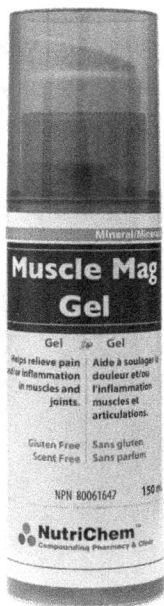

Sore muscles? Stiff joints?
Loosen things up using our
topical magnesium gel!

Purchase this product at www.nutrichem.com

NutriChem™
Personalized Health Solutions

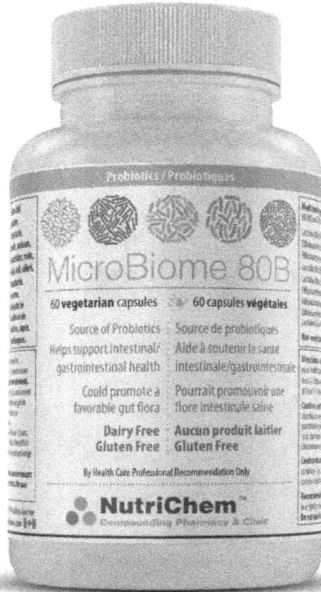

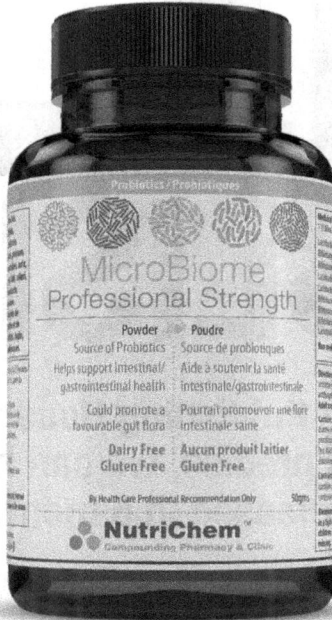

Balance YOUR Microbiome
like a professional!

Purchase this product at www.nutrichem.com

NutriChem™
Personalized Health Solutions

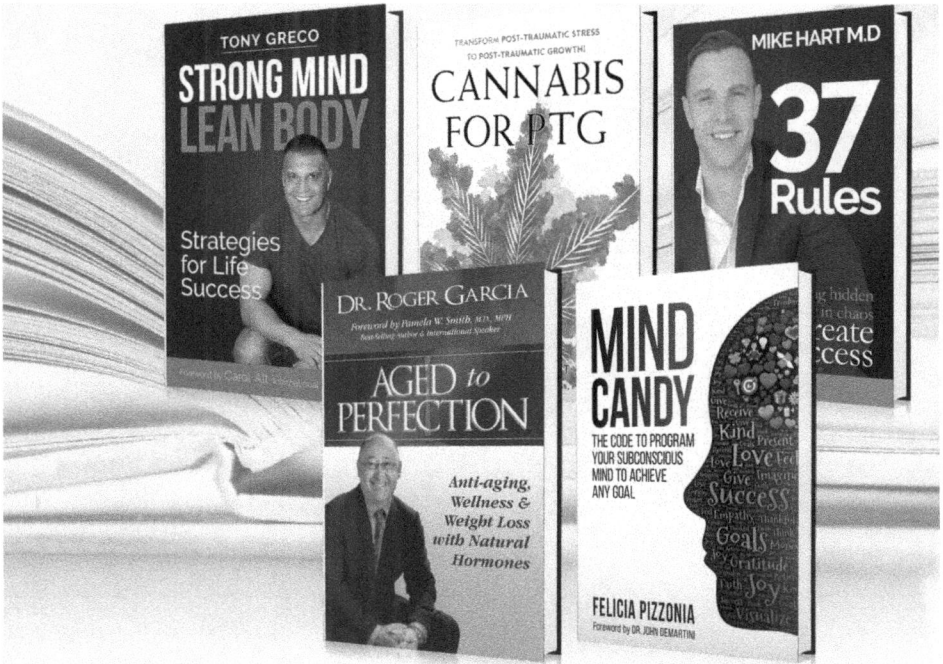

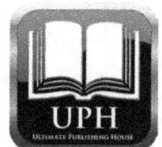

www.ingramcontent.com/pod-product-compliance
Lightning Source LLC
Chambersburg PA
CBHW050239270326
41914CB00041BA/2043/J